The Elemental Cleanse

28 days to a healthy body, calm mind, and awakened spirit

PAMELA QUINN

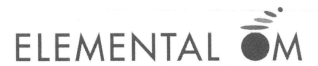

Requests for permission should be addressed to:

Elemental OM Permissions Dept.

9510 Montgomery Road, Cincinnati, Ohio 45242

email: info@elementalom.com

www.elementalom.com

ISBN-10: 1477646701

EAN-13: 9781477646700

Library of Congress Control Number: 2012911346

CreateSpace Independent Publishing Platform

North Charleston, South Carolina

Thank you to my yogis. Your dedication to self-discovery inspires me.

What People Are Saying About
The Elemental Cleanse:

Dr. Patricia David

"As a physician with a focus on proactive, preventative medicine, I am always looking for ways to help patients take control of their health while minimizing the use of prescription medications whenever possible. The Elemental Cleanse is the perfect adjunct to virtually every health management regimen; instead of offering "magic" potions or quick fixes, Pamela's program teaches people how to manage food, physical activity, and bad habits in order to achieve optimum health.

The Elemental Cleanse also gives people a road map to a clear, calm, positive mind—perhaps the biggest factor in achieving overall good health.

As a participant in The Elemental Cleanse, I can honestly say that Pamela's personalized support, lessons, detailed explanations, and gentle nature make the program fun, easy to follow, and truly enlightening.

After the twenty-eight days, I now see myself and the world in a different light; I have not felt this good, and this happy, for over a decade.

Knowledge really IS power—and this program is truly different because it doesn't just put a Band-Aid on your health problems. Instead, The Elemental Cleanse helps you get to the root of your issues so that you can finally make a real change in the health of your body and mind."

~ DR. DAVID

I Feel Giddy

"Physically, I feel better than I have in at least seventeen years. Mentally, I was depressed and now I am not. I actually feel giddy at times. I have really missed that side of me."

~ D. F.

In Control of Sugar!

*"My weight loss goals were met, **fifteen pounds in thirty days** is significant. I am now in control of my sugar habit."*

~ B. B.

Week 2 of The Cleanse

*"This Cleanse is amazing; even though I am not behaving perfectly, I have lost six to eight pounds and am **forming new, permanent lifestyle habits**. I now realize more what I should and should not eat. Priceless!"*

~ Privacy Respected

Create Positive Change

*"The Cleanse is an amazing experience. **It can change your life** in ways you weren't anticipating. I highly recommend this to anyone who is looking to feel better."*

~ J. L.

After One Week

*"I've slept for **eight hours or more three out of four nights this week!** I'm keeping track of when I feel tired during the day, but ultimately, I've already noticed a difference in how I feel. I'm not so exhausted all the time."*

~ A. H.

So Much More

"The Cleanse was everything Pam said it would be and so much more. I have known what to do to be healthy, but I am DOING it. I am taking the time to take care of myself."

~ P.Y.

I Made Some Very Necessary Changes That I Thought I Was Not Strong Enough to Do

"Before I did the Cleanse I had some bad habits that I let happen every day without even thinking about them. I was very unhappy with myself for my weight, drinking, and eating bad. The Elemental Cleanse has helped me make some very necessary changes that I thought I was not strong enough to do."

~ Jennifer

The Lifestyle Reset That I Needed

"The Cleanse was wonderful! It was the lifestyle reset that I needed. I feel so energetic. I feel that I'm glowing again. I have lost six pounds and that was not even a goal of mine. I feel fit and healthy again. I feel very connected to the path that I had lost sight of and am motivated."

~ Kim

The Best Thing I Have Ever Done for Myself

"I am fifty-five years old and have always taken self improvement seriously. The Elemental Cleanse is the best thing I have ever done for myself. It truly embodies the concept of holistic care. Pam is a natural leader and very down to earth. She will help you look at and question your lifestyle. Ayurveda is all about balance and this program is a great way to begin to see the possibilities of your potential."

~ Mary Beth O.

I Had Hit Rock Bottom

"I didn't feel loved. I was depressed. I am now able to feel again. I'm able to show compassion. I moved out some negative things and replaced them with positive things. As a result, I no longer have that heavy feeling about me. I allowed myself to open up and allow things to happen to me. I started to manifest. I stopped trying so hard. I just allowed myself to be. I now know and understand when I'm trying and when I'm being. It makes a HUGE difference."

~ Joy

Post Cleanse

"I am three months post-cleanse and on the eating plan. My cholesterol has dropped forty points and I've lost a total of twenty-five pounds since starting the class in May."

~ A. P.

My Skin Is Clear

"I lost eleven pounds, several inches, my skin is clear, and my hair is a little stronger. I found that I felt very calm and content throughout the majority of The Cleanse."

~ S. R.

Contents

Introduction

"Suffering needs no introduction."

$\sim$ Pamela

Never before has there been such an immediate need for a holistic modality to facilitate emotional, physical, and spiritual health. As a society, we are plagued by disease, weight gain, and stress. There exists a myriad of short-term solutions addressing the symptoms of our dysfunction, but few of these solutions go to the heart of suffering and facilitate real and permanent healing.

Welcome. You are about to embark on a twenty-eight-day physical, emotional, and spiritual journey known as The Elemental Cleanse. I created this program more than four years ago and have taught it to hundreds of people in person. The results have been so good that I have passionately committed myself for the last year to get the program in book form and make it accessible to the masses. Of course people have lost weight, but that is not the reason I created this program. I created it as a means by which to introduce people who have never heard of the science of Ayurveda to this holistic and beneficial lifestyle.

I learn by doing. This Cleanse is a full immersion into healing on every level: physical, emotional, and spiritual. If you suffer from weight gain, fatigue, inflammatory conditions, irritable bowel syndrome, arthritis, stress, insomnia, depression, lack of vitality, or just overall lack of joy, you will benefit from this program.

My Journey and Inspiration

My gift is that I have been blessed with a spiritual education that resulted from a debilitating back injury. In May of 2002, I woke to the worst pain of my life. My entire back was in spasm. I could barely move. I received physical therapy for one year. My first exercise was to simply lie on my back and hold my belly in. I couldn't even lift my legs. For that year I lived on muscle relaxers, Valium, sleeping pills, and loads of alcohol. I got really depressed. I had never experienced chronic pain or the deep, dark depression that comes with it. It consumes you, and it destroys everything. It hurt to put my shoes on. It hurt to unload the dishwasher. I could only drive when I wasn't loaded on muscle relaxers. My daughter was three at the time, and I would go to the swimming pool with her just to hold her. My marriage quickly started to decay as my (now ex-) husband grew impatient with my depression. I was miserable.

After a year of therapy, I was still in pain, but at least I could function. I went to yet another doctor, who simply told me that there was nothing wrong with me and I would have to learn to live with the pain. At the time, I thought he was the worst doctor ever, but as it turns out he was an angel in disguise. You see, 90 percent of back pain is psychosomatic (in your head).

Everyone always asks me what I did to hurt my back. I usually joke that I rearranged all the furniture in my sleep, because the truth is I didn't do anything. I simply woke up unable to move.

If you were to look at the circumstances of my life at that time you would be shocked to discover that I wasn't happy. I was a stay-at-home mom to two awesome kids. I lived in an eight thousand square foot home on a golf course with crystal chandeliers and all the "fixins." My AmEx had no budget. I had a white minivan, a convertible sports car, and even the requisite golden retriever. If you looked at my life, you would think I had it all. I was living the American dream.

I think it was George Carlin who said they call it the American dream because you have to be asleep to believe it.

My American dream came with a husband who I perceived as critical and controlling, not only of my actions, but also of my appearance. My American dream didn't include the fact that I love to work and needed to work to feel fulfilled. My American dream didn't include my connection to Spirit, which has been with me my whole life and was tucked away because it didn't fit in with what I knew from society.

That final doctor freed me from my dream by telling me there was no hope for me. I knew at my core that was wrong. I went home, threw out all of my drugs, including the anti-depressants, and went to work healing myself. I had heard that meditation could ease back pain, so I bought a book about meditation. If I'm going to do something, I like to do it right, so I signed up for meditation classes and a seven-day retreat. I met many spiritual healers at my retreat. I had no idea that these people even existed. My mind began to open as I realized there are so many ways to heal and receive Spirit.

At my retreat, we practiced very gentle yoga twice a day. We ate Ayurvedic food. We meditated. I started to feel so good. When I returned home, I found a yoga studio near my home and went five days a week. After five months, I was pain-free. My meditation practice was tough. The first three months of it I simply sat down twice a day and cried. I called it "scheduled crying." I had a lot to process. My father was a very dark man…an alcoholic whose alcohol consumption fueled destruction all around him. He left when I was thirteen. My mom never recovered. I felt abandoned and alone at a very young age.

Additionally, I was in the process of having to make some very tough decisions about my marriage. I felt alone in my marriage, and this feeling was intensified by the chronic pain and depression I was living with. All of this I simply processed for the first three months of my meditation practice, and then I finally did meditate. I started to change my life and heal on every level. I made those tough decisions to end my marriage, expand my education, and even start a business of my own helping and serving others…doing what I love.

My life has changed so much since I began living a yogic lifestyle. I wake up with gratitude pretty much every day. I still have problems come up, but I've learned to stay centered through them. I'm still changing and expanding. Each year brings some aspect of my being to explore. I feel young, vibrant, and capable of accomplishing anything. I have no fear. I've learned to love myself and be kind to myself. I no longer have the husband or the lifestyle, but I still have the kids and the golden retriever, and I love them in a much healthier way.

This practice works. I have to share it with as many people as possible because I know that it can help and heal them. I love to see people shift and grow. There is always a moment when I am teaching this program, usually week 3, when I will see a light turn on in someone's eyes. I will see them light up with hope. Everything about them in that moment changes as they suddenly realize that they are coming up for air. It's beautiful. I want to see people shift every single day. I can't even describe it adequately. When I see them heal, it heals me too. That's the real reason I do this.

Thank you for letting me be part of your transformation. Enjoy the journey.

Namaste,
Pamela

Namaste *means "I honor the place in you in which the entire universe dwells. I honor the place in you, which is of love, of truth, of light and of peace. When you are in that place in you and I am in that place in me, we are one."*

Before You Begin

The Elemental Cleanse is taught by Pamela in person and online at *www.elementalcleanse. com*. If you would benefit from personal support, additional verbal guidance, and motivation, check out Pamela's teaching and coaching schedule at *www.elementalom.com* as well as the online version of The Elemental Cleanse.

Plan to give yourself some time to read the first two chapters of the book and to gather the suggested materials and get organized. The Cleanse is designed to be completed in twenty-eight days, but many participants empower themselves to spend more time in each week and experience a slow cleanse.

Carefully review the section on herbal therapy and determine if the herbal kit is right for you. The herbs do facilitate elimination of toxicity in your system. I highly recommend that you take them as part of the Cleanse if you can. The section explaining the herbal kit outlines the beneficial effects. Everyone can perform the sesame seed oil massage, so you should plan to purchase a bottle of organic sesame seed oil as part of your preparations even if you decide you cannot take the herbs. All herbal and oil therapies needed for Cleansing can be purchased at www.elementalom.com.

Ayurveda

You are about to undertake a twenty-eight-day journey to a healthy body, calm mind, and awakened spirit. The Elemental Cleanse is founded in the traditions of Ayurveda, a system of holistic living and medicine that originated in India many thousands of years ago. The word *Ayurveda* translates to "the knowledge of life." It is a systematic science that utilizes the natural rhythms of nature to prevent, diagnose, and treat disease. It is also a philosophy and spiritual tradition honoring the idea that the human experience is one of body, mind, and spirit. This spiritual tradition is the Vedic religion. A sage called Veda Vyasa in texts that date to 3000 BC captures this spiritual tradition. The texts are called the Vedas. The Vedas are written in a language called Sanskrit. Sanskrit is the oldest Indo-European language and is a seed language for our modern languages. You will learn a little bit of this sacred language during your Cleanse. Your first word is *Ayurveda*.

The four books of the Vedas cover all topics of living, including health, spirituality, self-realization, astrology, herbal therapy, gem therapy, color therapy, yoga, mantra, surgery, business, government, and even the art of war. One book, the Rig Veda, is the basis for modern day Ayurveda and yoga. Other books have birthed from the Vedas. The oldest medical book in the world is called the Atreya Samhita. It is a compilation of all the Vedic scriptures that directly speak to the practice of Ayurveda.

The influence of Ayurveda can be seen in all the world's holistic medicine. Scholars from all over the world, including China, Greece, Italy, Egypt, and Persia, came to India to study this spiritual medicine. The father of Western medicine, Paracelsus, studied Ayurveda in the sixteenth century.

Two brilliant Ayurvedic physicians, Charak and Sushrut, condensed the original and complete knowledge of Ayurveda. There are now three main Ayurvedic texts, which are believed to be over twelve hundred years old—the Charak Samhita, the Sushrut Samhita, and the Ashtangha Hridaya Samhita.

Currently, Ayurveda is the most widely embraced preventative holistic medicine in the West, thanks to the fact that Ayurveda embraces new medicines and technologies. The Ayurvedic view is "if it is working for you, then stay with it." If you are controlling sleep disorders, depression, high blood pressure, or any other ailment with Western drugs, you should take the advice of your physician. Once you embrace the preventative and healing nature of this lifestyle, however, you will discover that you have no need for many of your prescriptive medications. If you want to stop taking any of your medications, do so with the guidance of your physician, as many do have side effects. It is an eye-opening experience to have your blood work taken before and after the Cleanse. In fact, one participant lowered her cholesterol by forty points! You and your doctor will both be amazed by the twenty-eight-day transformation.

Ayurveda is a simple science for life that teaches and empowers the individual to reconnect with the rhythms of nature. Ayurveda honors that you are naturally affected by the rotation of the planets, the pull of the tides, the changing seasons, and the movement occurring throughout your day in each minute. It honors that you are unique. It honors that you are a creature of this earth as well as of the divine.

It is profound what was known five thousand years ago. It was known that the Earth is round and rotates on an axis. It was known that the Earth traveled around the sun. Ayurvedic physicians knew how to diagnose and "treat" diabetes. The Indian physician Charaka called diabetes *madhumeha*. This translates to "honey urine." Ants and other insects were used to diagnose the disease. The bugs would be attracted to the sweet of the urine. Both Susruta and Charaka identified two types of diabetes, noting that the first appeared in younger patients and the second appeared in heavier patients.

Ayurvedic physicians also knew how to deliver complicated births. They even performed surgeries. More fundamentally, a plan for living that prevents disease, aging, and needless suffering was devised.

How did they know all of this without the use of telescopes, microscopes, and modern technology? The legend of Ayurveda is that great seers and sages of India known as Rishis received the teachings of the Vedas from the universe. Rishis are legendary yogis thought to have magical powers known as Siddhis and believed to live for hundreds of years. Imagine an aging man sitting in a loincloth on top of a mountain in the snow meditating in perfect peace and physical comfort. These men sat in meditation and asked God, the universe, the cosmic mind, or their higher selves many of the same questions we ask ourselves today. Why am I here? What is my life's purpose? How do I stay healthy, vibrant, and young? It is believed that through the meditation process, the Rishis received from cosmic consciousness the formula for living a healthy and happy life. This formula was passed down for generations in prose and finally captured in the Vedas and, around 500 BCE, in two medical texts called Susruta Samhita and Carkaka Samhita. The formula identifies the building blocks of nature, and indeed the whole universe, as five great elements: Space, Air, Fire, Water, and Earth. This formula explains how to use the elements to prevent, diagnose, and treat disease.

I don't know if it is true that the Rishis received this information in meditation or not. I guess it seems kind of far out. Perhaps these Rishis of five thousand years ago were simply great observers of nature. Perhaps they simply sat by their fires and noticed that when a log is tossed onto a fire it transforms to ash. Maybe they then had the thought, "Wow, that's just like when I eat, it goes in one way and comes out another. Perhaps I have fire in my belly."

Maybe they watched a dry, dead leaf blowing on a fall breeze and observed that the leaf would quickly dart one way, then another, and finally come to an abrupt halt, only to fly up again.

Perhaps they had the thought, "Wow, that's just like my mind. My thoughts go this way and that and suddenly stop. I must have wind in my mind."

Perhaps they observed the mountains and noticed that the mountains never changed. Maybe they were surprised by the consistency of the trees and plants to return to flower each spring. They paused to think that the bones, the muscle, and the fat of their bodies appeared slow to change, just like the mountains. They could count on this consistency. Perhaps their bodies were made of the same earth as the mountains. It's really a very elegant and accessible way to identify with our bodies and minds.

Ayurveda teaches that all disease stems from poor digestion—of food and of thoughts. Your liver is the foundation for your physical digestion, because it is a vital part of the digestive process. It has more than five hundred thousand functions and can largely be thought of as the "oil filter" for your body. It filters up to two quarts of blood each minute. The liver transforms food into nutrients that feed your cells. It builds metabolic enzymes. It breaks down hormones, converts vitamins and minerals, and produces bile, cholesterol, estrogen, and immune substances. It stores blood and glycogen and regulates blood sugar.

It is believed that due to poorly functioning livers, we suffer from arthritis, heart disease, cancer, hormonal imbalances, depression, anxiety, suppressed immune function, and weight gain. Thyroid function is directly linked to the liver.

The liver's job is to analyze every single thing that you put in your body. It decides if the substance is toxic or nontoxic. This includes analyzing not just food, but also atmospheric toxins such as cigarette smoke and other chemicals. It also includes viruses, parasites, fungi, allergens, and unhealthy bacteria.

If your liver is overworked because of the pollution you are consuming, it will not filter as efficiently and you may suffer from high cholesterol, aches and pains, acne, psoriasis, allergies, fibromyalgia, PMS, mood swings, sluggishness, depression, bloating, weight gain, high blood pressure, constipation, and much more. The Elemental Cleanse focuses on nourishing the liver and getting it back to maximum functionality. All the cells of your liver are replaced every ninety days. That means that you receive a new liver every ninety days. The next twenty-eight days are going to begin a new growth process for a healthy and healed liver.

If you are unable to appropriately discern your thoughts, feelings, and personal beliefs, you will suffer from poor digestion in your mind. You will struggle in your relationships, in your job, and during your alone time. Drama and unhealthy habits will rule your life. You will never realize the life of your dreams, the life that you know is waiting for you to begin.

I believe you are here to live a healthy, happy, enriching life full of love. The Cleanse will give you the toolkit and the fresh start you need to achieve it. Let's begin by understanding the foundation for all of creation, the five great elements.

The Five Great Elements

All things existing on the material level are made from some combination of the five elements. They are the building blocks of creation. The five great elements are Space, Air, Fire, Water, and Earth.

In Ayurvedic terms, Space is the element that contains everything. Space, unlike the other elements, does not change. It is the one constant in your body and your environment. Space in your body does not go out of balance. It is a consistent aspect of your nature; it is your spirit.

Space is holding material existence together.
Its job is to "contain or limit expansion."
You cannot affect Space through your thoughts, words, or deeds.
It is cold, light, and dry.
The sense of sound or hearing is associated with this element.
In the body, it is the empty space between your molecules and your thoughts.
On a quantum level, we are empty space.

Space (Ether or Akasha) is the foundation of the other elements. Perhaps it's the vastness of the night sky when looking up that makes me think that there is something around us that is holding all of this together. In science they call the space between *dark matter* or *dark energy*. This is because our scientific measurements use the speed of light as a constant. Because there is no light, science hasn't quite figured out this energy.

There is some disagreement in Ayurveda what element was first. Some will argue that it was the Earth element, others Space. I believe it was Space because Space to me seems like the most intimately connected to Spirit. When you look to the properties of Space and Spirit, they are similar. Both are holding you together. Both cannot be changed by you, and both are simply a consistent presence regardless of what you are going through or choosing. This makes me think of the nonjudgmental and ever-present nature of Spirit.

I also think it is fascinating that Space is associated with sound. The Bible tells us that the universe was created with a "word."

By the word of the LORD were the heavens made; and all the host of them by the breath of his mouth. For he spake, and it was done; he commanded, and it stood fast. ~ *(PSALM 33:6, 9)*

Yogis will tell you that the universe was created with a "sound" called the vibration *aum* or *om*. AUM or OM is a Sanskrit letter. It is deemed to be the most powerful sound of the Sanskrit alphabet.

OM,
The imperishable sound, is the seed of
All that exists
The past, the present, the future—
All are but the unfolding of OM
And whatever transcends the three realms of time,
That indeed is the flowering of OM.

~ *UPANISHADS*

For the purposes of Cleansing, you do not need to know a thing about this element other than its properties, which are cold, light, and dry. You were born with a certain amount of Space in your body and mind, and there isn't anything you can do to change or affect it. Space in your body is simply the empty space between allowing for flow and communication. Space is the inside of your mouth, your nose, your lungs, your gastrointestinal tract, and your abdomen.

To deepen your intellectual, physical, and emotional attachment to space, plan to go outside tonight and stare at the moon and the stars. Notice the space between and imagine what it would be like to be floating in space just like an astronaut. I'm sure you will imagine that it is very cold, light, and dry. I'm sure you will be stunned by the vastness of space.

"To look out at this kind of creation and not believe in God is to me impossible."

~ Astronaut John Glenn

Water is the element of love.
Its job is to nourish.
Water is very difficult to affect. It is stable.
It is cool, smooth, nourishing, moist, and oily.
The sense of taste is associated with this element.
In the body it is the plasma, blood, mucus, and saliva.

Water (Jala or Apa) is the element of love. It is nourishing, soothing, and calming. Without adequate water supply, the human body starts to die within three days. Without the sensory stimulation of taste, touch, movement, and smell to stimulate the release of serotonin in the developing brain of an infant, a baby may grow to be a person with depression or violent and antisocial behaviors.

Water is a very stable element. There isn't too much you can do to personally affect this element in your body other than to drink too much or too little. Salt intake directly affects this element. Maybe you have had the experience of bloating after you have indulged in salty snacks like French fries or potato chips. The bloat is a response to balancing the water content of your body. Water in your body is the liquid plasma, urine, sweat, and saliva.

For purposes of the Cleanse, you need to know how to drink for your body type. You will take the quiz in just a bit to determine your body type. How much to drink will be discussed in Week 1 of the Cleanse.

Air or Vayu is moving everything.
Its job is to expand.
It is moving, unpredictable, cool, light, and dry.
The sense of sound or hearing is associated with this element.
In the body and mind, it is any moving function like
thinking, speaking, breathing, and eliminating.

When I think of the Air element I always think of a fall breeze. It brings with it a sense of excitement. It energizes you, it's fresh and makes you want to try something new. Think back when you were a child starting school. It was a time of excitement as you embarked on a new year of education. The rhythms of your family life changed as new routines were established.

The breeze is unpredictable. It gets strong and then softens. It blows up and then down. It suddenly stops and just as suddenly starts again. The breeze brings a chill and makes you want to snuggle and dress warmly. Standing in the breeze for a long time can exhaust you, especially if it begins to blow hard.

In your body, the Air is all that is moving. It is the movement of the lungs in respiration, the act of thinking, of swallowing, of eliminating, and of nerve impulses.

Sit quietly with your thoughts for a few minutes and notice how they move like the Wind.

Fire or Tejes is transforming.
Its job is to create change.
It is hot, bright, intense, and abrupt.
The sense of seeing is associated with this element.
In your body and mind, it is your ability to discern and decide.
It is transformation in your body; digestion and fighting infection.

When I think of Fire, I always think of a bonfire. It is hot, intense, and bright. It snaps and crackles and in a way talks back to you. It is abrupt, suddenly flaring up and then calming again. Fire holds your attention. Its intensity is mesmerizing, and you find yourself staring into its light. You are drawn to the flames.

When the Fire has done its job on wood, the wood is left transformed. In your body, Fire regulates the body's temperature, digests food, and absorbs and assimilates hormones, enzymes, nutrition, and your thoughts. The light of the world is taken in through the Fire of your eyes.

Sit quietly for a minute and imagine yourself in your last moment of anger. Did you suddenly erupt? Did your body become hot? Did you begin to sweat? Now let that thought go as well as the stressful situation.

Earth or Prithivi is grounding.
Its job is to create stability.
It is cold, dense, heavy, and slow.
The sense of smell is associated with this element.
In your body and mind, it is your larger mass: bones, muscle, fat, and cartilage.
It is your memories, your compassion, and your love.

When I think of the Earth, I always think of a boulder sitting in a shaded forest. The boulder has a little bit of moist moss growing on it. The boulder is heavy and dense. You push, but it won't budge. You touch it, and it is cool.

If you were to sit down on the boulder, you would feel very secure and grounded. It never appears to change. You could walk by it every single day for twenty years and it would appear the same. All changes are happening so slowly you wouldn't even notice. In your body, the Earth gives you the same structure, stability, and strength. It is also what gives you stamina. Imagine if you got the boulder rolling down a hill—it would be very hard to stop. In your body it is your bones, teeth, muscles, fat, and skin.

Go outside and pick up a stone or, better yet, sit on a boulder! Notice how it makes you feel very connected to the Earth. Notice its soothing and nurturing energy. In Greek mythology, the Earth goddess is called Gaia. She is mother earth. Mother earth was born from what the Greeks call chaos and what yogis call Space. Mother earth gave birth to all the other gods and goddesses.

You are now familiar with all five great elements, Space, Air, Fire, Water, and Earth. Spend some time this week in nature. Go for a nice, leisurely walk and simply observe the quality of your surroundings. Stare into the vastness of the night sky. Experience a sense of wonder in your mind. Sit by a stream or pond and appreciate the calm that settles in your body and mind. Smell the breeze. Does a feeling of anticipation percolate inside of you? Light a candle and stare into its flame. Notice how you relax and don't want to stop staring. Is effort required to break your gaze? Take your shoes off and sink your toes into the grass or dirt. Close your eyes and feel the nourishing coolness. Lie down in the grass, close your eyes, and feel the support of the earth beneath you.

Now it's time to find out what proportion of these elements are found in your body and mind. We will take two simple quizzes, one for the body and one for the mind.

The Element Quiz

On the day of conception, the way you think, the way you look, and the way you metabolize were determined. This is your constitution, or, in Sanskrit, your *prakruti*. You are as unique as the pattern on a snowflake. Just as all snowflakes are made from water, so too are all humans made from the elements, Space, Air, Fire, Water, and Earth. Just as no two snowflakes are alike, so too no two humans are alike. In fact, you could meet all seven billion people currently residing on this planet and you would never truly find your twin.

Because of your unique constitution, you respond and react to situations, events, food, drink, and medications in a special way. For example, many people eat tomatoes or pasta sauce and experience heartburn or indigestion. Why? Many people take prescription drugs with no side effects, but one in a thousand will end up at the emergency room at the hospital. Why? Many people simply go with the flow and suffer little from stress. Others respond with anger or anxiety over the smallest of things. Why?

The reason is that they have different amounts of the elements in their mind and body. You may be a person who has a predominance of Space and Air and just a touch of Fire, Water, and Earth. Or you could be a person with a predominance of Fire, a touch of Water and very little Space, Air, and Earth. You may have more Earth, a little bit of Water and very little Space, Air, and Fire. Each of these people will display different characteristics that make up his or her personality and physical structure. Each person will respond differently in similar situations and each will digest his or her food differently. All contain all the elements, just in a different proportion.

The quiz you are about to take is designed to help you understand what elements are predominant in *your* mind and in *your* body. We test for the elemental composition by testing for the actions or forces of the elements. Each element, alone, does nothing. It simply exists. The elements combined, however, create forces or tensions. There are three forces in your body: Vata, Pitta, and Kapha. These forces are called *doshas.*

Let's think about the properties of the elements for a moment and reflect on how they differ. Let's take Space and Air. Space has the job of containing everything. Air has the job of expanding. A person with a lot of Space and Air contains two elements that are polar opposites in action. Space wants to hold tightly, and Air wants to expand. A tension exists between the two called Vata, and this tension keeps them playing nicely. A person containing a lot of Fire and Water also has two elements that oppose. Fire wants to transform and Water wants to soothe. Too much Fire will evaporate Water. Too much Water will put out Fire. A tension called Pitta builds to keep the two from destroying each other. A person with a lot of Earth and Water has two contradicting elements. Earth is stable and inert. Water is fluid and mutable. Earth wants to stabilize Water, and Water wants to move the Earth. The tension of Kapha keeps them in harmony.

These forces affect thought, speech, sleep, hunger, emotions, and metabolism. Living in harmony with these forces creates a balanced and peaceful existence. Thoughts are clear, intentions are known, and your body is healthy, vital, and free of disease. When these forces take over your mind or body, however, you become unbalanced. You may begin to suffer sleepless nights, racing thoughts, depression, lethargy, anger, anxiety, weight gain, and even serious illness.

Depending on the predominance of the elements in your body and mind, one or more forces will exhibit most strongly. This is your *dosha,* or your first response in any given situation.

The Doshas

Vata or The Wind (the elements of Space and Air are abundant): When you think of Vata in your body or mind, you have only to think of the fall breeze. The breeze is cool, crisp, and light. It is erratic with no apparent reason for blowing or routine. It brings freshness, energy, and a feeling of something exciting to come. Vata in your mind is your thoughts. It is the gift of creativity and inspiration. Vata in your body is the force of movement, talking, swallowing, and eliminating. Vata creates a person with a thin frame, irregular eating habits, and quick speech. It creates a creative person with invigorating speech and an energetic and adaptable mind.

Pitta or The Fire (the elements of Fire and Water are abundant): When you think of Pitta in your body or mind, you have only to think again of the bonfire. The bonfire is hot, bright, and pungent. The fire can flare up quickly to amazing intensity and then settle abruptly. The fire transforms all that it consumes. It radiates power, force, and energy. Pitta in your mind is your ability to process emotions and ideas. It is the gift of discernment. Pitta in your body is the force of transformation; digestion, fighting infection, and sight. Pitta creates a person with a strong build, strong digestion, and precise speech. It creates a bright and warm person full of charm with high intelligence and good discrimination.

Kapha or The Earth (the elements of Earth and Water are abundant): When you think of Kapha in your body or mind, you have only to think again of the boulder sitting in a cool forest covered in moss. The boulder is heavy, dense, and cool. It does not change quickly; it is strong, stable, and inert. The boulder sits calmly through the shifting of the forest. Kapha in your mind is your ability to remember and feelings of compassion and understanding. It is the gift of love.

Kapha in your body is stable, lubricating, and predictable. Kapha creates a person who is heavyset with smooth skin. It creates an easygoing, thoughtful, and caring person who is devoted and loving.

Who you are, your constitution (prakruti) does not change. You will take the test and discover your dosha. This is your dosha for life. This is who you are. It is your first response.

The word *dosha* translates to "that which goes out of balance." This means that you always have to maintain the balance of your doshas because the balance changes minute to minute. Think about how quickly anger can flare up. Anger is an out of balance expression of Pitta (The Fire). Think about the last time you couldn't fall asleep because your thoughts were racing or you were worried. This is an expression of Vata (The Wind) running wild. Think about your last day as a couch potato. That is Kapha (The Earth) sucking you into the mind-numbing escape of TV.

To live a harmonious, balanced life, you must become aware of your first response in your body and mind and how to maintain balance.

Taking the Quizzes

Take the Body Element Quiz and the Mind Element Quiz to find out what your first response or dosha is. This will give you insight into the way your mind and body behave.

Take your time filling out the tests, but don't dwell on the answers. If you struggle to answer any question, remember that your first thought is usually correct. If you are still uncertain, ask a friend to give you the answer. If you are *still* uncertain, choose The Wind (Vata). People who change a lot, change quickly, and have much unpredictability in body and mind tend to be The Wind. Also, people who have a hard time deciding tend to be The Wind.

When you take the quizzes, imagine a time of your life when you felt good, vibrant, and healthy. I find that many people have been living out of balance for so long that they don't know how they feel anymore. They can't even remember feeling good. Don't worry. At the end of twenty-eight days, we will revisit these quizzes again. You will be back in balance and then you will have a much clearer picture as to what dosha you are.

You will notice that the quizzes are separated between your mind and your body. It is very common to have one predominant dosha in your mind and another in your body. Sometimes they are the same, but not always. The purpose of The Elemental Cleanse is to help you to feel the energies of the doshas in both mind and body. I separate mind and body to simplify the teachings of Ayurveda. Many other Ayurvedic books and websites do not. I find that this confuses people when they are first introduced to Ayurveda and makes living an Ayurvedic lifestyle harder to understand. Simply allow this Cleanse to be an experience of the doshas. Once you begin to balance and resonate with your prakruti, you can dive deeper into Ayurveda.

Most people will take the quizzes and find that they have two predominant doshas in their body or mind. This is normal, and it is actually a very good thing, because it gives you more stability and less chance of going out of balance. Don't let this confuse you. We are going to have a tangible experience of the doshas, and by the end of the Cleanse you will know what is "in play" in your body and mind.

Have fun and don't judge yourself while taking the quizzes. I find that we instinctively want to resonate with what is perceived as a "more favorable" quality. Remember that you, like the entire universe, are a broad spectrum of all emotions, and this includes admirable qualities like compassion, generosity, and understanding. It also includes troubling qualities like lack of follow through, criticism, and laziness. I promise you, if you were only the positive qualities on that spectrum, you would be the most boring person on the planet. The combination of all qualities creates a dynamic personality.

The Mind Element Quiz

Your Mind: What Is Your Dosha?

Circle the element that best describes you. If you simply can't decide, choose The Wind (Vata). This quiz determines the predominant element or dosha in your mind.

Sleeping Patterns:
I sleep very lightly and awaken easily. (Wind) ✓
I fall asleep easily and sleep for a moderate period of time. (Fire)
I sleep very deeply and for long periods of time. I love to nap. (Earth)

Sleeping Patterns:
I have a hard time falling asleep. (Wind) ✓
My biggest worry that keeps me from sleeping is work-related. (Fire)
I have very few sleep problems other than sleeping too much. (Earth)

Dreams:
I dream a lot. My dreams are vivid and active. (Wind)
I do not remember my dreams well. My dreams are vivid
and full of passion. They frequently involve chasing and negotiating. (Fire) ✓
My dreams are peaceful. I remember them. (Earth)

Speech:
I talk quickly and a lot and have a hard time staying focused. (Wind) ✓
I speak with precision and I love a good debate. (Fire)
My speech is slow and deliberate. I think before I speak. (Earth)

Shopping:
I'm an impulse shopper. I love to buy little gifts for people. (Wind) ✓
I tend to indulge in very expensive, high-quality items when I do spend. (Fire)
I shop to "buy" happiness. (Earth)

Climate:
I love it sunny and warm. I do not like to be cold. I hate drafts. (Wind) ✓
I prefer cooler weather. I can become irritable when it is hot and humid. (Fire)
I prefer a warmer temperature. Cold and wet make me achy. (Earth)

Movement:
I'm like a butterfly flitting from activity to activity. (Wind) ✓
I move with purpose. People notice when I enter a room. (Fire)
I have a very relaxed and fluid gait. (Earth)

Organization:
My home or office may appear messy to others, but I know
  where everything is.   (Wind) ✓
I like a well-organized environment. I have a place for everything.   (Fire)
I am a collector of things. Sometimes I accumulate clutter.   (Earth)

Work Preference:
I love the activities of creation such as brainstorming and conceptualizing. (Wind)
I like to be in a leadership position. I do not like working
under someone. I am a visionary and strategic planner.   (Fire)
I like a routine to my job. I prefer to work for others and
treat my place of employment as "family."   (Earth) ✓

Moods:
I'm moody.   (Wind)
I have a very strong, determined, and stubborn nature.   (Fire)
I am emotionally sensitive and very caring for others.   (Earth) ✓

Stress Response:
When stressed, I become anxious and worried.   (Wind) ✓
When stressed, I become short-tempered, irritable, or critical.   (Fire)
It takes a lot for me to stress, and then I tend to shut down.   (Earth)

Focus:
I have a hard time paying attention. My mind wanders.   (Wind) ✓
I am focused and able to pick effectively through information.   (Fire)
It takes me a long time to take in information, but I never forget.   (Earth)

Forgiveness:
I get over things pretty quickly. Forgive and forget.   (Wind)
I can sometimes be revengeful, jealous, or self-centered.   (Fire)
I tend to hold onto hurts. It takes me a long time to release hurt or pain. (Earth) ✓

Add up the circles by Wind, Fire, and Earth. The one you have the most of is your dosha.

The Body Element Quiz

Circle the element that best describes you. If you simply can't decide, choose The Wind (Vata). This quiz determines the predominant element or dosha in your body.

Frame:
I tend to be thin.   (Wind)
I have a medium build and tend to have a more athletic structure.   (Fire)
I have a heavy build and am strong.   (Earth) ✓

Weight Gain:
When I gain weight, which is hard to do, it tends to settle on my belly.   Wind)
I can gain and lose weight easily.   (Fire)
I gain weight very easily and lose it with difficulty.   (Earth) ✓

Bones:
If you were to hug me, you would feel my skeletal structure.
My bones are brittle and fragile.   (Wind)
I am well-proportioned and tend toward an athletic build.   (Fire) ✓
My bones are heavy and larger.   (Earth)

Skin Condition:
My skin tends to be thin, dry, rough, and cool.   (Wind)
My skin is fair and tends to have issues: rashes, acne,
blackheads, whiteheads or, blotching.   (Fire)
My skin is pale and smooth with very few marks.
My pores are almost invisible.   (Earth) ✓

Nails:
My nails tend to be dry, brittle, or flaky.   (Wind) ✓
My nails are strong and flexible.   (Fire)
My nails are strong and thick.   (Earth)

Menstrual Cycle (for women in child-bearing years; all others simply skip):
My periods tend to be irregular. I don't bleed a lot and it tends to be
    dark red. I get really bad cramps and sometimes constipation.   (Wind) ✓ ?
I have regular periods, with a heavy flow that is bright red.
    I feel like my periods last an extended time and I may experience
    mild cramping and loose bowels.   (Fire)
My periods are regular with a light, average flow. I experience
    bloating and mild cramps during my period.   (Earth) ✓ ?

Appetite:

My appetite is irregular. I may go all day without eating and not realize it. (Wind)

My digestion is very strong as well as my appetite. I like routine meals
and get grumpy if I don't eat.   (Fire) ✓

I have a stable appetite. I can skip meals.   (Earth)

Cravings:

I love salty, crunchy snacks.   (Wind)

I crave iced beverages and cold food.   (Fire)

I crave sweets and starches.   (Earth) ✓

Digestion:

My digestion is unpredictable. I can be normal, be constipated, have diarrhea,
or experience gas and bloating from day to day.   (Wind) ✓

I have strong digestion. When I do have issues it tends to be heartburn,
indigestion, or loose bowels.   (Fire)

My digestion is slow and steady. Food feels heavy in my belly. (Earth)

Temperature:

My hands and feet tend to be cold. I tend to be cold overall.   (Wind) ✓

I tend to be hot.   (Fire)

My skin is cool to touch, but I do have cold hands and feet.   (Earth)

Total your circles. The element circled the most is your dosha for your body.

You may have struggled with the body portion of the dosha quiz. Many people do so because they have been living out of balance for a very long time and don't really know the answers anymore. Don't worry. We will take this quiz again at the end of the Cleanse, and you will better understand which element resonates with you after you come back to balance. Just like with the mind, you may find that two or more elements describe you almost equally. All of the doshas are present in your body, and it's quite common to have an even split between two. Less common is to have the doshas split almost equally between all three, but it does happen.

Interpreting Your Element or Dosha Quiz

Now that you have completed your quiz, you are aware of the predominant elements in your body and mind. The combination of the five elements in a person's body and mind establish as doshas or energies of the body and mind. An abundance of one or more elements in comparison to the other elements gives a person a predominant dosha, or way that the body or mind responds or reacts. The doshas express the qualities and characteristics of the elements. Each person's dosha is unique and every individual has a personal formula for balance.

It is interesting that the Sanskrit term *dosha* translates to "that which goes out of balance." Living with a balanced dosha creates health. The purpose of the Cleanse is to bring your doshas back to balance.

You may be surprised now that you have taken your quiz that the predominant doshas in your body and mind do not match. You might be surprised that some of the doshas were very close in score. You may find that you have a Wind (Vata) mind and an Earth (Kapha) body. You may have a Fire (Pitta) mind and a Wind (Vata) body. You may have both a Fire (Pitta) mind and Fire (Pitta) body.

It gets confusing quickly. Don't worry; you will understand this easily in the end.

Mind	Body
Wind	Wind
Fire	Fire
Earth	Earth
Wind	Fire
Wind	Earth
Fire	Wind
Fire	Earth
Earth	Wind
Earth	Fire

The most confusing outcome is to have two columns on either the mind or the body test that are almost matching in score. You look at the test and think, *My body has the most Wind, but it sure has a lot of Fire in it too. Which one am I, really?* The same can be true for the mind as well.

In Ayurveda, this is known as duo-dosha, or two doshas. This is actually more the norm than not. Regardless of your predominant dosha, you have all three doshas in your mind and body. If you strongly relate to two doshas, it simply means that both sets of characteristics are present. This actually gives you a much more stable structure that is less likely to go out of balance. The challenge is to figure out which one you more strongly resonate with to maintain balance.

Some participants will have the experience of having three doshas. This is called tri-dosha and is not very common. These people have a very stable constitution, but when they do go out of balance it is harder for them to come back to balance.

For purposes of the Cleanse, simply pick the digestive system that you most strongly relate to and create consciousness around that. Other body characteristics such as the hair, nails, and skin can be explored later.

The Wind has delicate and variable digestion. You may find that you do not experience intense hunger and you often skip meals. You crave salty snacks. You may experience lots of allergies and sensitivities to food. Your digestion tends to run dry toward constipation, but it is also erratic. One day you may be loose, one day dry, and one day normal. The Wind has a hard time gaining weight and when it happens, the weight settles on the midsection and is mostly due to poor routine and impulse eating.

The Fire has strong digestion. You experience intense hunger for breakfast, lunch, and dinner and find that you become grumpy if you skip a meal. You like to eat at the same times each day. You find that you can eat almost anything. If anything does bother you, it tends to be spicy or sour foods. When your belly is upset, you tend to become loose during elimination and have heartburn, indigestion, or an acid belly. You can easily gain and lose weight. When you do gain weight, it is because of overindulgence and it settles evenly on your body.

The Earth has stable digestion. If anything, The Earth may become a little bit sluggish at elimination. You love food but can skip meals with little effect. You crave sweets and really have to watch yourself to not eat too much of them. You have probably been fighting your weight since childhood and easily gain weight while struggling to lose.

After completion of this course, you may be aware of and able to identify with the following statements about you:

Your digestion is strong like FIRE.
Your thoughts are unpredictable like WIND.
Your skin is creamy, smooth, and free of pores like the EARTH.

I could go on endlessly naming all parts and functions of your mind and body. That's how incredibly complex you are! You can see that this can easily become confusing. I recommend you simply accept your dosha. For the next twenty-eight days, learn about your dosha, but follow the instructions for Cleansing. Cleansing is intended to bring all doshas back to balance and is a methodology. When you finish Cleansing, you will take the dosha quizzes in a balanced state, and you might find that you may pick different answers. Many people taking the Cleanse have been out of balance for a long time and really struggle to pick quiz answers because they are so out of touch with who they really are.

Explore the extended recommended reading list, but don't confuse yourself in the details, because for the next twenty-eight days it doesn't matter what your dosha is. That's right. *It doesn't matter until the end of the Cleanse.* I can't stress that enough. Don't go there yet. You will become confused and fall off your Cleanse without intention. You will learn routine and diet for your dosha after you have cleansed. At that point, your dosha becomes important.

For the next twenty-eight days, you are here to cleanse your body, mind, and spirit of accumulated emotional and physical toxins. This plan is an elegant system of cleansing for all doshas. At the end of the Cleanse, we will go more in-depth. By then you will have experienced and learned so much that it will be effortless. You will know all the doshas and how they feel in your body and mind.

SPECIAL NOTE

During the course of your Cleanse, you may experience some specific situations because of your predominant element. Some examples of common situations include the following:

I am losing weight and that is not my intent. I am the Wind body type. What should I do?
I am not losing weight fast enough to satisfy me. I am the Earth body type.
The potent spices like garlic and pepper are irritating me. I am a Fire body type.
I cannot sit still to meditate. I am the Wind mind.

These situations and many others are addressed at www.elementalom.com. I've been administering the program for many years and have been thorough in anticipating these situations. If you do not find your particular situation addressed at the website, please e-mail your concern to *pamela@elementalom.com*.

Let's have a little bit more fun with the mind body types to help you begin to understand your nature. Again, this is for fun. *Do not* attach to it.

The Wind or Vata

The Wind Mind

The Wind is the tension created when the elements Space and Air combine. This dosha in Ayurveda is known as Vata. You do have the other doshas, Fire (Pitta) and Earth (Kapha), in your mind; however, their expression is not your first response.

To understand how your mind behaves, you only have to think of the elements that combine to create Vata: Space and Air are dry, rough, cool, light, penetrating, moving, broad, unlimited, and unbounded. Think of a cool autumn breeze. The breeze blows every which way and suddenly stops. It is unpredictable and may just as suddenly start moving again. There is no rhythm or routine to the movement. The breeze brings with it a sense of excitement and change.

You probably exhibit the following characteristics in your personality:

- We all have Wind in our minds. It is the activity of thinking. Combine that with a predominance of Wind (Vata), and you have a person who does a lot of thinking. Even in a balanced state, your mind tends to go and go and jump from thought to thought. This can be wonderful because The Wind mind is very enthusiastic, lively, energetic, and creative. However, it can be troublesome, too, as you may find that your sleep is interrupted even when you are totally living in balance. You dream a lot of vivid dreams. You are intuitive.

- Because of your active mental state, you are prone to anxiety and worry. You may find that you worry about absolutely everyone and every possible situation, including much about life that is completely out of your control. The lesson for The Wind is to surrender to outcome and stay in the present moment.

- You probably love all things new. You are familiar with the top ten books on the best-seller list, you know the latest headline news, and you are signed up for a class in the latest trendy fad. You know a lot of people and have a large circle of friends. You have excellent short-term memory. You love to shop and spend and pick up lots of small little treats for yourself and friends. It is a challenge to save money.

- You can be easily distracted. In fact, you may be reading all ten books on the best-seller list at the same time. You may find it hard to finish any one of them, and you may not retain the story very well. While you are familiar with the latest headline news, you may not exactly understand the history or geography of the world's events. You are a big-picture person. You tend to jump from job to job, so while you are a jack-of-all-trades, you may not be a master of any one. Your circle of acquaintances is wide, but you may have few close friends. You can appear aloof, and you may struggle to listen to others.

- Your imagination and creativity make you an entertaining person. In fact, The Wind is usually the life of the party. Quick-witted and able to out-think most others, you generate laughter and excitement. You are the person who picks others up. In fact, your strong intuition knows when others are a bit down and you are always quick to lend a smile, hug, or laugh to shift the energies of others.

- You are fabulous at finding creative solutions to problems. In fact, you would thrive working in a job where you initiate creative solutions. You don't necessarily want to be in charge of others, but you do like to have freedom of movement and freedom in how you spend your time. You lack follow-through, and finishing projects may be difficult. Surround yourself with people who can take your fabulous ideas and see them to fruition.

- You are very sensitive. Others may not realize how deep your feelings truly run, and you may find that you are easily hurt. You hate making mistakes and worry that what you do is never good enough. Sometimes you feel scattered. You will find that you need long periods of rest and silence each day to soothe your nerves and nourish your sensitive heart.

The Wind Body

The Wind body is more of an ectomorphic body. You are tall or short with a slender build. You do not exhibit strong muscle development. You have good flexibility. You tend to have low levels of fat and low body temperature that should be monitored. Yoga and gymnastics are wonderful for you because of your light frame.

- You tend to be a cold person and may even wear sweaters in the summertime. You suffer in the cold and wind and should take precautions to always dress warmly and cover your throat, face, and head.
- You have dry skin, nails, and hair. You are probably prone to flaky skin, especially around the nose and mouth. Your nails may be brittle and peel or flake. Sesame oil is your best friend. Use it morning and night, rubbing it into your nail beds and soaking your hair weekly overnight.
- You have a delicate digestive system that suffers from dryness. You may find that you are sensitive to foods and do not have a strong appetite. You skip meals and do not notice that you are hungry. You snack on and crave salty, crunchy foods. You may suffer from constipation one day and be regular the next day and loose the day after. Your digestion is unpredictable. Routine eating of warm and nourishing foods is key to your digestive health.
- When a person with a Wind body moves, it is quick and unpredictable. You may have a hard time sitting still and find that you talk with your hands and are quite animated. You work in bursts of energy and find that you burn out quickly and must rest.
- The instability of your system also means that you have very unpredictable immunity. You probably get sick often, picking up every little bacteria or virus that comes your way. This is due in part to the dryness in your body, but also to your lack of routine, which impairs your digestion. Never forget that the strength of your digestion is directly linked to your ability to fight disease.

Some famous Wind bodies include Nicole Kidman, Kate Hudson, Keira Knightley, Gwyneth Paltrow, Adrien Brody, Orlando Bloom, and Jim Carrey.

The Fire or Pitta

The Fire Mind

The Fire is the tension created when the elements Fire and Water combine. This dosha in Ayurveda is known as Pitta. You do have the other doshas, Wind (Vata) and Earth (Kapha), in your mind; however, their expression is not your first response.

To understand how your mind behaves, you only have to think of the elements that combine to create Fire: Fire and Water. Fire is hot, bright, intense, and abrupt. Water is cool, smooth, nourishing, moist, and oily. Your personality exhibits these qualities. You probably exhibit the following characteristics in your personality:

- The Fire in all minds is the process of discernment. Combine that with a predominance of Fire (Pitta) and you have a person who is very good at making decisions, managing others, and leading. In a balanced state, this is a person who is "large and in charge." You are a dynamic speaker, leader, and motivator. Even in balance, this can also be troublesome, as you may find that you take on the problems of the world and the responsibility to solve them.

- Because of your determined mental state, you are prone to suffer from work-related stress. You may find that you feel you are the only one who can do things the correct way and that those around you are not as intelligent or capable. The lesson for the Fire is to learn to delegate through leadership and to allow others the freedom to be who they are.
- You stay focused. Fires have incredible follow-through. You don't necessarily want to do the work of completing a project, but you like to see a project through from start to finish. Fires have the ability to plan long term and love goal setting.
- You are fabulous at leading others to do tasks. In fact, you would thrive in a job in which you are in charge of others. Fires suffer enormously when working for a company or boss who micromanages. If working for another, Fires need to be empowered and set free to make decisions and follow through. Only someone who you greatly respect and admire and from whom you can learn will lead you.
- You take care of others. Fires are passionate about family, friends, and the world. You see yourself as a humanitarian and wish to solve problems for others. You are self-reliant and rarely ask for help from others while constantly offering it.
- You can be reluctant to share your emotions and fearful that the emotional ups and downs in life are a sign of weakness. Others may not realize how badly you are hurting, as you are very good at masking your pain. You hate mistakes and perceive that they are the fault of others' incompetence. You prefer to do everything yourself so that it is done the "right" way. Sometimes you feel very stressed by the heavy load of responsibility you carry. You will find that you need periods of intense physical activity followed by rest to release your stress. You crave nature, especially water.
- You probably love your routine and are disciplined and organized. Fires like their offices and homes to be neat and organized. Fires tend to get up and go to bed at the same time each day as well as eat meals in a routine fashion. Fires can be vain and are disciplined in their physical practices, gravitating toward energy-releasing activities such as running, hiking, biking, and weightlifting.
- Fires are good with money. When purchasing, a Fire will go for the big-ticket item that is luxurious.
- Fire minds tend to have very passionate and active dreams.

The Fire Body

The Fire body tends to be more mosomorphic. This means that you have a wedge-shaped body (think about the V that a body builder makes with his torso). Arms and legs are muscular, shoulders are broad, and hips are narrow. The body appears narrow from front to back, but not from side to side. There is a minimum of fat on the body.

- The Fire exhibits a lot of strength, agility, and speed. You are athletic and probably love cardio and lifting weights. You see immediate benefits from these sports. It is very easy for you to gain and lose weight.

- You tend to be a hot, meaning that you are sensitive to heat and sun, with skin that tends to burn and freckle. Use sunscreen and minimize your exposure to the sun and to extreme heat. Your skin tends to feel hot, and you may sweat a lot. The heat annoys you.

- Your skin tends to be oily and is prone to outbreaks, even when in a balanced state. Stress really does a number on your skin. Your hair may be thin and accumulate oil.

- You may have a stronger body odor and breath. When you consume heating foods such as onion, garlic, and peppers it is more noticeable than for the other body types.

- You use your life force up more quickly than the other elements. Because of this, you are prone to premature aging and graying. Your hair may thin at an earlier age as well.

- You have very strong digestion and can eat pretty much anything you want to. If you put on a few pounds, it's easy for you to take them off. The caution for The Fire is not to overindulge. Because you can eat pretty much whatever you want and easily lose weight, you tend to overdo it. No one needs to tell you to eat three meals a day. Your friends could set their watches by your hunger, and if you are not fed you may become grumpy and irritable.

- If you have any digestive discomfort, it is in the form of heartburn, indigestion, sour belly, and loose elimination. Your emotions strongly affect your digestion as well as any hot or spicy food.

- You tend to have a nice asymmetrical athletic build and you love to exert yourself, so it's no problem for you to exercise vigorously. Be sure not to overindulge in exercise as well. It is very common for Fire types to want to lift weights and artificially inflate their bodies. Make sure to incorporate a nice cool down after your workouts.

Some famous Fire bodies include Julianne Moore, Debra Messing, Jennifer Aniston, Madonna, and Cindy Crawford. Famous men include Tom Cruise, Matt Damon, Denzel Washington, Justin Timberlake, and Kobe Bryant

The Earth or Kapha

The Earth Mind

The Earth is the tension needed to allow Water and Earth to combine. This dosha Ayurveda is known as Kapha. You do have the other doshas, Fire (Pitta) and Wind (Vata), in your mind; however, their expression is not your first response.

To understand how your mind behaves, you only have to think of the elements that combine to make the force of the Earth: Earth and Water. Earth and Water are heavy, cold, soft, lubricating, sweet, stable, immunity-enhancing, and slippery. Envision a boulder covered in a bit of moss sitting in a cool forest. The boulder is a constant, and if you were to walk by it every single day, you would not notice that it is changing in any way. If you were to lean against the boulder, you would find it to be cool and grounding at the same time. Its solid, unmoving presence is calming and nurturing.

You probably exhibit the following characteristics in your personality:

- The Earth in all minds, regardless of the predominant force, is what gives a person stability, compassion, and love. Combine that with a predominance of Earth (Kapha), and you have a person who is grounded, nurturing, and stable. When I think of my Earth friends, I think of the people I go to when I simply want a shoulder to cry on or someone to make me feel at home. The Earth is the nurturer in all of us.

- Because of your stable mental state, you are prone to being very laid back. You take things in stride and don't obsess or worry very much. In fact, you can be a little too laid back and often don't effectively deal with situations. Many Earth types will shut down or seclude if life gets a little too stressful. You may even seclude on occasion when you feel you simply can't deal with what life is handing out.

- You may appear stubborn to others. It takes a very long time to come to decisions. You simply do things in your own time and take the time to absorb information and choose. The Earth tends to do everything a bit slower, including reading, but has amazing long-term memory.

- You probably love all things that are of family and that have a story. You are the person in the family who creates the photo albums and hangs onto report cards, old records, and your grandmother's recipes. You remember history and love to share all the memories of childhood and family vacations. You are very attached to your family and will adopt anyone into your family, including your friends and coworkers. You like taking care of them and showering them with love and affection.

- You are focused and love routine. The Earth enjoys doing the same things each day. You are a person who loves to have a nine-to-five job that is stable and predictable. You are a long-term employee. You are attached to your employer and coworkers. You may choose to stay in a job that you have grown out of due to the feeling that the company needs you. In fact, you love that your desk has been in the same spot for many years and would be unsettled if it were to move. You get attached to objects and may accumulate clutter at work and at home.

- You are fabulous at finishing projects and following through. You take great pride in your work, your dedication, and your loyalty. Your friends, family, and coworkers know that they can depend on you.

- You are caring. You love to take care of others and give abundantly of yourself. You must be cautious not to give all of yourself away. The Earth has incredible stamina, and you will suffer greatly in situations that no longer benefit you. The deep sense of caring and obligation can be overwhelming to the point that you have trouble making life decisions.

The Earth Body

The Earth body is more of an endomorphic body. You may have shorter arms and legs and a larger frame and mass. Your arms and legs tend to accumulate more fat. Your bones are larger and heavier. Your muscles are larger. You are prone to excess weight and weight gain. It is imperative that you have invigorating daily movement or the weight will not stay off. If you cease your daily movement, you can easily lose conditioning that you have worked so hard to achieve.

- While you are not a "cold" person, your skin tends to be cool to the touch. It may even feel moist. You probably suffer in cooler weather and should take precautions to stay warm.
- You are a cuddly, soft person. Your skin is soft, your hair is soft, and your body stays soft and pliable. You have very good flexibility with loose joints. Earth types are easy to identify by simply touching their smooth, pore less, and utterly soft skin.
- You may be prone to excessive mucus and bloating. The recommendation for The Earth is to drink when thirsty but not to drink excessively, or you will suffer from bloat.
- You are sweet. Sweet is one of the six tastes of Ayurveda. We will learn about this a bit later, during the Cleanse. Just know for now that our average American diet contains a lot of this taste, including pasta, breads, meat, dairy, fruits, and sweets. You have a lot of this taste in your constitution, so you really shouldn't eat much of it.
- The Earth is very stable, meaning it is slow to change. It probably takes you a while to get going in the morning. If you fall into an energy slump, it may take a while to turn that around as well. The good news is that this stability translates into forward momentum once you do get going. An Earth body committed to a movement practice will get into a good routine and stick to it.
- When a person with an Earth body moves, it is slow, steady, and graceful. Dancing is one of the most positive activities for an Earth body.
- The stability of your system also means that you have a strong immune system. You probably don't get sick very often. The caution is that you may be so stable that you push yourself even when you are feeling run-down or even sick. The Earth body needs to rest when it is feeling run-down.
- Your digestion tends to be reasonably good, and you can skip meals with no problem. Your digestive disorder tends to be that your digestion can become sluggish and it may take time to eliminate. You must stoke the digestive fire with spicy and cooked food.

Some famous Earth bodies include Marilyn Monroe, Catherine Zeta-Jones, Queen Latifah, Beyonce, Oprah Winfrey, and Kate Winslet. Famous men include Antonio Banderas, Shaquille O'Neal, Tom Hanks, and Dan Rather.

I still don't really get it. What is my predominant element?

I get this comment a lot. You've filled out your quizzes, but you don't really feel like the person that the quiz says you are. Let me give you a few anecdotal examples. Please note that because these are meant to entertain I take full license to exaggerate and, hopefully, not offend, so that you will remember.

The Dinner Example

The Wind:

If the Wind mind shows up at a dinner party, she will probably be late or early. If she brings a dish to share, it will be a recipe that she has never tried before. Otherwise, she may simply not bring one or might quickly grab something at the store on the way. The Wind will quickly charm and delight all of your guests. As the hostess, be sure to seat her strategically around the Earth minds, because she will really pull those folks out of their shell. The Wind will lead the conversation with current events, esoteric thoughts, and all of the craziness that she has gotten into in the last week.

The Fire:

The Fire type will definitely be at your party if he said he would be. He will likely be on time or might strategically arrive glamorously late. The dish that he brings will be hot and spicy and elegantly presented. The Fire type will jump into the kitchen and help you start organizing your dinner. When the dinner bell rings, the Fire will usher the others to the table. The Fire's warmth and charm will make him a popular person to be seated next to. The Fire is likely to listen to the conversation and fill in the holes with important points and information. The Fire is likely to go back for seconds and will probably organize the cleanup for you.

The Earth:

The Earth type will call in advance to offer to help you with your party. You may decline, but she will show up anyway in loving support. When the soufflé burns, call the Earth and she will improvise a dessert for your party. The Earth will bring a sweet, yummy treat to share. It will probably be from her grandmother's collection of recipes kept after her grandmother passed on. At dinner, you might find her to be shy and quiet. However, she will surprise you at the end of the meal by making the most profound comment about the evening's conversation. The Earth will stay in the kitchen after the dinner, cleaning and putting everything away, while you continue to mingle with your guests. When the party is over, The Earth will still be there to make sure that you had a great time and to see if you need to talk through any of the events of the evening.

The "Almost" Car Wreck

The Wind:

Imagine that the three different types are almost in a car wreck. *Almost* is the key word here. The wreck never happens.

The Wind takes full blame for the incident. She becomes very anxious and worried. Her racing thoughts will sound something like this, "Oh my gosh, I can't believe I almost smashed into the back of that little old lady. What would happen if I hurt her? Does my insurance cover her and me? Did I pay my insurance premium this month? I can't even remember the name of my agent—I should put that in my phone. What if I would have gotten a ticket? My rates surely would have gone up. I need to shop my insurance. This car is getting old. I should get new tires. Who would I have called to pick up the kids from school if I had to go to the hospital? I wonder what the best hospital is…blah, blah, blah." Sadly, the Wind will still be talking about this nonevent to herself and others at day's end.

The Fire:

The Fire immediately blames the other person. Think road rage. Colorful language and hand gestures may follow the angry glare. A brief synopsis of how bad every other human on the planet drives may follow. The Fire will let it go after all the steam is blown off.

The Earth:

The Earth is immediately grateful that the accident did not happen. Probably the Earth wasn't even driving. She was sitting in the back because her go with the flow nature doesn't need to be in charge. The Earth won't think about the situation again other than to comfort the anxious Wind or the angry Fire who was driving.

Hunger

The Wind:

The Wind tends to lack routine and that includes eating. Winds frequently skip breakfast and maybe even lunch. It isn't unusual for The Wind to pause around 2:00 pm and wonder if she has eaten that day. She will actually have to think about it to determine that she did or didn't. By time she arrives home, The Wind is famished and will snack on salty crackers while preparing dinner. Dinner arrives, and she finds she is full. Late evening snacks of popcorn and chips are normal.

The Fire:

The Fire needs to eat. This person wakes up hungry and has breakfast, lunch, and dinner around the same time each day. If you have ever been shopping with a friend who has become irritable as the noon hour comes and passes without food, you were probably shopping with the Fire. Simply feed the Fires in your life. They need to eat. The Fire type craves spicy food. It isn't unusual to find the Fire standing in the fridge with the door open and eating out of a jar of banana peppers. Of course, this also gives him heartburn and indigestion.

The Earth:

The Earth loves food. She loves the colors, the textures, and the smell and is quite colorful in her discussion of food. She is very aware that every single thing she puts in her mouth goes straight to her hips. An Earth friend of mine used to say that she couldn't walk by a tray of cookies without wearing them home on her backside. You get the point. Earth craves sweet treats and will often turn to food in times of crisis. Emotional eating is a characteristic of The Earth.

Have fun with your elements. You can see from these anecdotal illustrations that it can be fun and entertaining to learn who you are. As you learn to recognize the doshas in others, you'll have greater insight into how they operate. I think the most magical part of knowing a person's nature is that you can respect and honor who they are and release any desires you have around wanting them to change. The Wind will always be a little messy, a little distract-ed, and a little late. The Fire will always be large and in charge, a little critical, and probably more right than wrong. The Earth will always be slow to change, slow to get moving, and your best friend.

How do the doshas go out of balance?

The Wind (Vata) Leads...

Learning to recognize and manage when the doshas in your body are going out of balance is very important for maintaining short-term and long-term health. If you are empowered to quickly respond to the initial onset of imbalance, you will sustain good physical and mental health.

You can take a quick look back at your element quizzes to remind yourself of the predomi-nant force in your mind and in your body. This is your true nature, or first response. In Ayurveda, remember, this is termed *prakruti*. As a reminder, you have all the elements in your mind and body as well as all the forces (doshas). One is predominant, and it is your instinctive nature to behave with its properties. This is important because depending on your predominant element you may be more likely to experience certain disorders.

Regardless of your predominant element, the forces behave in the following way: The Wind (Vata) is always the first to go out of balance, The Fire (Pitta) is always the next to become ag-gravated, and finally The Earth (Kapha) goes out of balance. Everything follows The Wind (Vata). It leads.

Read the Following Carefully and Twice...It's Profound

Ten percent of our health care dollars are spent on 90 percent of disease. Ninety percent of disease is caused by out-of-balance Wind (Vata). Examples include the initial onset of cold, headaches, backaches, general aches and pains, constipation, and sleep disorders. These are easily treated with routine and nutrition. You don't have to go to the doctor or pharmacy and spend money to remedy these conditions. Now think about the fact that The Wind always leads the other doshas. If you could stop the imbalance in the Wind, you wouldn't have to worry about those other diseases. Simply knowing when your Wind is going out of balance and knowing how to ground it would prevent denser diseases like diabetes, heart disease, cancer, arthritis, and depression.

So 90 percent of our health care dollars are spent on 10 percent of disease, and 10% percent of disease is related to The Earth (Kapha). Examples include diabetes, cancer, heart disease, arthritis and depression. When you experience these types of disorders, you must go to the doctor and the pharmacy. Typically you are in for a long journey through these diseases.

Many people take the balance quiz and become quite upset as they realize they have an overall imbalance. Please don't worry. The good news is that The Elemental Cleanse will quickly pull you back to balance in twenty-eight days. The Wind disorders will dramatically shift within the first two weeks. Any Fire disorders such as heartburn, indigestion, and skin irritations will shift by the third week and through the fourth. If you are battling an Earth disorder, this will take beyond the twenty-eight days to shift completely, but it will really start to move. An Earth disorder is weight gain. You didn't become overweight overnight, did you? Of course not. The Earth takes time to put weight on and time to safely take it off.

Situations by Element or Dosha

The Wind (Vata)

Dry skin, nails, and hair
Interrupted sleep
Insomnia
Constipation
Fatigue
Headaches
Intolerance to cold
Malnourishment
Anxiety
Worry
Racing thoughts
Loss of memory
Inability to focus

The Fire (Pitta)

Redness and rashes
Inflammation
Ulcers
Heartburn
Indigestion
Poor vision
Intolerance to heat
Premature graying
Premature baldness
Aggression (road rage)
Irritability
Impatience
Thinking you are right
Heart attack

The Earth (Kapha)

Sluggish digestion
Weight gain
Obesity
Sinus congestion
Asthma
Allergies
Cysts
Arthritis
Heart disease
High cholesterol
Depression
Inability to decide
Bloating

If you are experiencing any of the above situations, don't worry. At the end of the Cleanse you will be in balance and feeling great. You will have to continue to work on weight loss, high cholesterol, and the other chronic conditions by eating for your element or staying with the Cleanse eating plan.

The Balance Quiz

Let's take the Balance Quiz next to find out if you are in or out of balance. Answer the questions below, taking into consideration how you have been feeling for the past twenty-one days.

1. NOT AT ALL
2. LITTLE BIT
3. SOMEWHAT
4. MODERATELY
5. VERY MUCH

- I've been having trouble concentrating, I am forgetful.

- I have been talking a lot and having trouble listening.

- I have been having trouble sleeping.

- I have been very worried lately.

- I can't seem to stick to a routine. I am impulsive.

- **The Wind in Your Mind (total)**

- I have no routine. I eat, sleep, and perform activities at inconsistent times each day.

- I am suffering from gas and bloating.

- I have constipation. My elimination is hard and dry.

- I have been suffering from a lot of situations, such as back pain and headaches.

- My skin, nails, and hair feel dry.

- **The Wind in Your Body (total)**

- I have been very impatient lately.

- I am critical and judgmental.

- I have been very opinionated and forceful in sharing my opinion.

- I feel like others simply aren't doing a good job and I need to be in charge.

- I have been losing my temper.

- **The Fire in Your Mind (total)**

— My skin is suffering from outbreaks, rashes, and inflammation.

— I have heartburn or indigestion.

— I have hot flashes.

— I have loose elimination.

— My breath seems bad. My body odor is sour.

— **The Fire in Your Body (total)**

— I have been quiet and withdrawn. I do not want to deal with conflict.

— My thoughts are dull. I don't want to try new things.

— I feel jealous, possessive, and needy.

— I want to make changes, but just can't.

— I feel depressed.

— **The Earth in Your Mind (total)**

— I've been gaining weight and holding it.

— I feel sluggish in the morning and want to sleep in.

— I have sinus congestion, nasal allergies, or asthma.

— I am retaining fluids.

— I have cysts or other growths.

— **The Earth in Your Body (total)**

You have completed the balance quiz and now have an understanding of your current state of health. Any score of nine or below indicates that that dosha is in balance. This is an area that needs maintenance and little attention. If you have any scores that are between ten and fifteen, you are suffering an imbalance in that area. You probably have been out of balance for a little while. Any scores over fifteen indicate an imbalance that you have probably been experiencing for some time.

It is not uncommon to have multiple categories of imbalance. Vata is usually the first dosha to go out of balance, followed by Pitta and then Kapha. If you are experiencing multiple imbalances, it simply means that you really need the Cleanse. Please don't be hard on yourself for letting yourself go out of balance. Intend to do your work for the next twenty-eight days and you will be back in balance.

Over the years I have worked with hundreds of people. If you do your work, you will be back in balance. I have never seen a person who does the work of the Cleanse not shift.

Let's move on to getting organized for the next twenty-eight days. Organization and planning are critical success factors for the Cleanse. We will begin with a snapshot of your current situation and then move on to time management.

Getting Organized

Assessing Your Current Situation

Complete this exercise as a way of stepping back and looking at your current situation with a clinical and objective eye. This will add a little reality check to your Cleanse. It will also help you to set intentions for the next twenty-eight days. What do you really want to shift and where do you want to focus your attention?

I'll be honest with you. I give you *everything* to work on for the next twenty-eight days because I have lots of people taking the Cleanse for lots of different reasons. Some find that they attach to the food, some to the emotional work, some to the spiritual work, some to yoga, and hopefully all to meditation!

You will naturally gravitate to that which most heals you. I do hope that you put effort into all aspects of the Cleanse, because it does all work together. That said, this Cleanse is a foundation for a lifetime of work.

Physical Health

With an objective and nonjudgmental eye, analyze your current physical health. How do you feel when you arise in the morning? Do you have enough energy? Are you currently under the care of a doctor and are you in alignment with your treatment plan? Are there any medications that you are taking that you would like to adjust or wean from? Have you been suffering from any situation for an extended period of time and can you imagine life without this situation?

Relationship With Work

Are you happy in your current job? Do you feel financially, intellectually and emotionally fulfilled? Do you like the people that you work with? Do you look forward to working? Do you feel that you work too much or too little? If you could do anything with your life, what would it be?

Family Systems Information

Do you have a happy home life? Do you feel that you give and receive an abundance of love and affection? Is there anything in your family relationships that you would like to shift or change?

Spiritual Identity

What is your experience of God or Spirit? What is not your experience? What is your heritage? What beliefs does your family have that you question and what are your questions? What do you celebrate? What do you believe? When do you feel most connected with Spirit?

Current Eating Routine

Be nonjudgmental in answering the following questions. You want to step back and get a snapshot of your current choices.

- Do you cook?
- Do you enjoy the grocery store?
- How many times a week do you eat out?
- Are you currently dieting?
- How many meals do you eat each day?
- Do you drink caffeine, including coffee, tea, or soda? If so, how much?
- Do you smoke?
- Do you drink alcohol, and if so, how much each day or week? Please describe your typical food day during the week and during the weekend.

What are your goals for The Elemental Cleanse?

What would you like to experience that is different from what you are experiencing now?

Now that you have completed your assessment, step back and look at the big picture of your life as an observer. Do not judge yourself or become critical. Chances are this process highlighted some of the choices and situations that have resulted in your current state of imbalance. Perhaps some surprises even emerged. Intend to shift how you make choices and transform over the next twenty-eight days.

Make the Commitment

Please read and sign this agreement as a commitment you are making to and for yourself. If your resolve wavers, go back to this page and refresh your memory as to why you are undertaking this journey. Sign co4nsciously and send out a huge positive intention to shift.

I, _____, am making a commitment on this date_____, 20__ to focus on myself for the next twenty-eight days.

I intend to:

- Spend time in meditation each day. The first week will include ten minutes each day; the second fifteen minutes; the third twenty minutes and the final week will include two rounds of twenty minutes each.
- Follow the routine for eating.
- Follow the routine for living by nature's rhythms.
- Spend time in silence avoiding the media, TV, excessive talking, and crowds.
- Perform my self-administered oil massage with The Elemental Cleanse oil on a daily basis and pamper myself.
- Listen to the advice of my doctor.
- Follow The Elemental Cleanse herbal supplement plan.
- Stop taking all herbal supplements that have not been prescribed or suggested by my doctor.

Signed_____

Making Time for Yourself

"Just Say No"

During the next twenty-eight days, it is critical that you take time for yourself. This program is truly about being self-focused and self-centered in order for you to be focused and centered for the rest of your life.

Taking time for self-care seems to be one of the biggest obstacles I hear to successful completion of the Cleanse. Once you finish the Getting Started module, you may realize that you want to delay your start date by a week or so until you get your personal calendar under control. Many people do this and have wonderful results.

The first week of the program seems overwhelming to many people. That's because it is your "getting organized" week. You are stepping back and looking at the changes that need to be made, including the new routines that need to be incorporated into your life, and you may feel a little overwhelmed. This is normal.

There are many parts of the program that a) take no time and b) you are doing in some fashion anyway. They include the following:

- Spending time in silence. This takes absolutely zero time.
- Turning the TV off. This saves time.
- Establishing a routine for bathing, bedtime, and awaking. This will ultimately save you time and allow your mind to become more efficient.

- Meditation. The first week is just ten minutes. If you can't find ten minutes to sit down all alone, then you need this Cleanse more than anyone.
- Shopping. You have to go to the store anyway. Just get organized prior to your shopping trip with your lists and be prepared. Make shopping a joy. Your early bedtime with reading can be reading a recipe book.

Your Family

You cannot abandon your family or your duties. So discuss your needs with your family. Your family does not need to participate in your Cleanse. While it may seem daunting right now, it is actually very easy to cook one meal for an entire family that all, including you, can enjoy. You will find that you are making various whole grain, vegetable, and bean dishes that pair nicely with your family's desire for a filet mignon. You will simply skip the filet. Don't be surprised if your family embraces the new foods you are introducing. When I teach this program in person, participants always comment that their spouse is also losing weight.

Tell your family what you are doing. Tell them that it is very important to you and that you want their support. Explain your reasons for embracing this program. Perhaps you are tired, frustrated, unenthusiastic, depressed, or suffering poor health. Perhaps you simply want to lose weight; everyone always understands this. Tell them you need to heal so that you can be your best for them. Explain to them that you will be eliminating dairy, alcohol, caffeine, processed foods, and meat from you diet. Explain that they do not need to do this.

Ask for their help in creating a more calming and nourishing environment. Helping with chores, keeping the atmosphere neat and free of clutter, keeping TV time to their rooms or at a minimum, or even just turning the volume down a notch will all be appreciated. Let your house get modestly messy. I find that people waste a lot of time each day managing their household, only to have it a mess an hour later. It's okay to let the laundry pile up a bit. It's okay if everything isn't perfect. We will establish one space in your home to be your "Zen" space. Let's let the rest go a little bit.

Plan on saying the word *no* a lot. When the PTO calls for the bake sale, say no. When your sister calls for a babysitter, say no. I know this is hard, but you have to bank on all the things you have said yes to in the past and know that you will say yes in the future. This is your time now, and you deserve to heal, connect, and become clear.

We seem to live in a society obsessed with serving children. We run and drop and schlep and pick up. Every whim and desire is fulfilled. It's killing the parents. Get organized. Cash in on all the times you have carpooled. Tell your kids they can begin lessons in a month. Allow coaches to find other volunteers. It's just a month. If you have small children, engage a babysitter to allow you a little "me" time. Call in a favor from a sibling or a grandparent.

Your Job

You cannot quit your job. You may find that the Cleanse significantly shifts your job in the future, but for now you must be present. If there is a way to schedule a little time off during the next twenty-eight days, do take advantage. Many people schedule the final week of the Cleanse as a "staycation," and they absolutely love it. At a minimum, be prepared with the *no* word. When your boss asks you to be the cochair for the annual fundraiser, say no. If you have the option of taking on a huge project or not, say no. Do pause and ask yourself if you are doing things at work because of a real need or because of an inability to delegate or trust others. I find my Fire minds seem to be the ones who suffer from this the most at work.

You will be greatly rewarded in the future for the time that you take now to learn these new skills. The Cleanse will change how efficiently you think, manage, and process. You will realize that taking a little time just for you each day creates a more vibrant, creative and happy person that serves the whole world in a much more elegant way.

I have included weekly overviews at the beginning of each week. Copy the weekly highlights and the schedules for Week 3 and Week 4 onto your own personal calendar. For each week, you have a "week at a glance." Add items to your calendar to keep organized. When reviewing the calendar, do notice that Week 4 is about rest and relaxation. Week 4 is the perfect week to schedule time off of work, babysitters, an Ayurvedic massage and maybe some special treat like acupuncture. Plan well and take advantage of this week.

Calendar Highlights

Week 1

Meditate ten minutes each day
One vegetarian meal per day
Emotional work is to release the past.

Week 2

Meditate fifteen minutes each day
Two vegetarian meals per day
Emotional work is to cultivate the purity of the ego and soul and to begin the process of connecting to your heart's desires.

Week 3

Meditate twenty minutes each day
Three non vegetarian meals all week
Prepare for Week 4 by practicing your Cleansing Dish.
Emotional work is to refine your choice-making abilities and to connect to your life's purpose.

Week 4

Meditate twenty minutes two times each day, for a total of forty minutes.
Follow the Cleansing diet.
Write your story.

Herbal Therapy

A Cleansing Kit can be purchased at www.elementalom.com. The Elemental Cleanse is not dependent on the use of herbal therapy, special drinks, shakes, or foods. I do highly recommend certain herbs as part of your Cleanse, however, because they add value to the experience and help to shift some stubborn conditions. All the recommended herbs are traditionally used in an Ayurvedic Cleanse. Think of the herbal supplements as food. In Ayurveda, anything we put in or on our body is food. In fact, neem is commonly used to make tea and triphala is made from three Indian fruits.

Many people, however, cannot participate in the herbal therapy due to situations such as pregnancy, nursing, thyroid conditions, or blood-thinning medications. These people still have profound results. Do check with your doctor if you have any concerns.

Neem: The Most Powerful Detoxifier Used in Ayurvedic Medicine

I discovered neem at the age of thirty-two when adult-onset acne reared its ugly head. My neck and jaw line were covered in boils that would last up to six months. I picked at and aggravated the boils, which led to redness and scarring. I found myself at the dermatologist and even the plastic surgeon looking for a remedy. Antibiotics and creams helped a bit, but the problem persisted. It was horrible.

At that same time, I began studying yoga, meditation, and Ayurveda. I stumbled upon neem while doing some holistic research into acne cures. I immediately started using neem soap and neem lotion and ingesting neem in capsule form. Not only did my skin immediately start to heal, but the redness and scarring began to diminish as well. I've been using neem ever since. There are a few herbs I take daily, and neem is one of them.

In holistic medicine we advocate managing stress and eating a wholesome diet to prevent acne. Herbs are therapy, and many shouldn't be taken long term. I find, however, that my Fire (Pitta) skin is easily upset by the slightest stress, changes in diet, and my ever-shifting hormones. If you are a woman over the age of thirty-five you can probably relate. Neem is safe to take daily, and I recommend it not for just treating acne, but for any skin condition. It's a powerful anti-inflammatory, and I have seen incredible results from people taking it to heal arthritis, irritable bowel syndrome, and migraines.

Neem is a wonderful addition to the Cleanse. It is a tonic for your liver that facilitates digestion. It works to soothe your doshas and your nervous system. You will notice diminished aches and pains, your skin will clear, and you will feel good. Neem works to cleanse your cells of accumulated toxins. Neem is bitter. Think about when you bite into something bitter. Your reaction is to spit it out. While cleansing, you ingest neem (don't worry, you won't taste it) and it is taken into your cells. The bitter taste of the neem stimulates your cells to literally "spit out" the toxins. We add to this process our oil therapy and the cells get lubricated so that the toxins come out even easier. All of these toxins end up in your digestive system and are eliminated naturally through your bathroom ritual.

Caution: Neem is not for you if you are experiencing malnutrition, chronic illness, or pregnancy. The literature is mixed on whether nursing mothers should take neem, but I think it wise to err on the side of caution and not take neem if you are pregnant. However, the Cleanse is appropriate for pregnant and nursing women and may be one of the greatest things you can do for yourself and your growing baby.

WHAT IS NEEM?

The neem tree *(Azadirachta indica)* is a scrappy little evergreen native to India. It thrives in harsh conditions, including poor soil and high temperatures. Because of its healing properties, people are now cultivating neem outside of India, in Asia, South America, and Africa. In the United States, we are testing the growth of the neem tree. I'm crossing my fingers that they flourish. I have three neem trees planted in pots in my home and yoga studios. They flourish outside in the Ohio summers, but they must be brought inside in the fall. They do moderately well inside, but they seem to long for their native Indian climate. Still they survive, offering their leaves for tea and facials.

In India, the neem tree is considered sacred because of its miraculous healing properties. It has been used as a holistic medicine for 4,500 years. In India, it is used to treat or prevent intestinal worms, malaria, encephalitis, meningitis, scabies, fungi, smallpox, head lice, diabetes, epilepsy, ulcers, headaches, and fevers. More than six hundred million people use the branches of the neem tree as a natural toothbrush. Neem has been shown to be effective in reducing cavities and healing gum disease. I've been using neem toothpaste and an electric toothbrush for years, and my teeth are almost as white as many of my friends who use harsh chemical whiteners. Besides treating gum disease and whitening teeth, neem provides the following benefits to your body (your doctor will like this list):

Antiviral	Capable of destroying viruses
Antifungal	Able to destroy fungi
Antimicrobial	Able to inhibit or destroy the growth of disease-causing organisms
Antibacterial	Able to destroy or inhibit the growth of bacteria
Antipyretic	Able to lower body temperature or prevent or alleviate fever
Anti-inflammatory	Able to reduce inflammation
Anti-tumor	Able to reduce the risk of tumor growth
Analgesic	Able to relieve pain
Immune stimulation	Able to enhance your body's immune system
Alterative	Able to cure or restore health
Anathematic	Capable of expelling or destroying parasitic worms
Anti-emetic	Able to prevent or stop nausea or vomiting

Triphala, Known in India as "Three Fruits": Amalaki, Bibhitaki, Haritaki

Please be aware that you are taking a blend of triphala and guggulu for purposes of Cleansing.

Triphala is a classic Ayurvedic formula comprised of three fruits. Amalaki is a source of anti-oxidants and vitamins. Bibhitaki fruit augments levels of protein and good cholesterol in the body, and Haritaki is an anti-spasmodic.

Some claim that triphala has properties that aid in weight loss. While it is true that triphala has laxative properties and can assist in the weight loss process through balanced elimination, *triphala alone will not promote weight loss*. It can, however, boost digestive and intestinal health and will help with constipation, parasites, diverticulitis, colitis, gas, cholesterol, irritable bowel syndrome, and ulcerative colitis.

Triphala is an integral part of an Ayurvedic weight-loss program, but Ayurvedic weight-loss programs address all dimensions of your life, including sleeping, eating, eliminating, and movement.

Guggulu, or Commiphora Mukul

Guggulu is a resin from a thorny tree that is native to Northern India called *Commiphora mukul*. The resin of this tree has been used in Ayurveda for thousands of years and documentation of its use dates back to 600 BC. Like many herbs, guggulu grows easily in poor soil. Herbs are thought to be more powerful as they must struggle to survive, making them strong.

Guggulu is commonly used to treat high cholesterol, obesity, fibromyalgia, diabetes, arthritis, nervous disorders, myofacial pain, endometriosis, acne, gout, and rheumatism. Swished in the mouth, it is also effective for canker sores and gingivitis. It is very effective for those detoxing from a drug or alcohol addiction. Although guggulu does not aid in weight loss, in a 1999 study conducted by researchers at the University of Nebraska and Beth Israel Medical Center in New York City, people who took 750 mg of guggulu each day and did a combination of strength and aerobic training three times a week for six weeks lost an average of six pounds; those who exercised but did not take guggulu lost only one pound or less.

During the Cleanse, you will learn about the "tastes" of Ayurveda. There are six tastes that, when included in your meals, allow your body and mind to feel satisfied. Guggulu contains four of the six tastes, including bitter, spicy, astringent, and sweet. Bitter, spicy, and astringent are all very light and cleansing.

Guggulu does have other positive side effects, including strengthening your hair and nails and eliminating the dark circles under your eyes. Guggulu also may have less pleasant side effects to be aware of, such as headaches, nausea, vomiting, loose stools, diarrhea, belching, and hiccups. Most of these adverse reactions happen at much higher doses (6000 mg). If you find yourself experiencing any of these side effects in the first week, pause to ask yourself if it is related to alcohol, caffeine, or sugar withdrawal. Many people experience headaches as they eliminate these stimulants from their system.

If any of the following describes you, you should not take guggulu:

- You have thyroid disease (talk to your physician).
- You are taking blood-thinning medicine (for example, Anaprox, Naprosyn, Fragmin, Lovenox, and Coumadin).
- You will be having any type of surgery within the next two wee
- You are pregnant or nursing.
- Estrogen interacts with guggul. Talk to your physician if you have any to this hormone.

Yoga

During the Cleanse, you will experience yoga and daily walking. Search for a yoga studio close to your home or work and plan to attend three to five classes each week.

If you are new to yoga, do not begin with classes with the following labels: power, hot, Bikram, Ashtanga, or vinyasa flow—unless they specifically say they are for beginners. Instead, look for a studio that offers hatha, new to yoga, restorative, slow flow, and yin.

If you currently have a power or hot yoga practice, add gentle, yin, and restorative to your weekly routine and minimize your participation in power and hot yoga. Power and hot practices are very heating to the mind. The purpose of the Cleanse is to soothe and calm your mind. You do not want your yoga practice to interfere in this process. At month's end, you can go back to your regular routine if it still resonates with you.

I teach Hatha yoga at my studio. I love it because it is accommodating to all body and mind types. Explore this month! Commit to an unlimited yoga pass and go as much as you can. You will feel so good.

Do plan to walk thirty minutes each day. I suggest daily walking after meals. After you finish a meal, simply walk out the door for five minutes and then turn around and come back. This will get your thirty minutes in easily and will facilitate digestion. If you are focused on shifting weight, plan to walk for thirty minutes at a time. The walking does not have to be brisk. Simply get out and enjoy nature. Do walk outside regardless of the weather.

If you are struggling with an exercise routine or you just don't enjoy it, please give it up for the next twenty-eight days. This may include running, biking, weight-lifting, aerobics, or pilates. On the other hand, if you do any of these and the exercise sends you into blissful state of mind, then please continue to enjoy your workouts. I find that many people are pushing themselves through workouts that they simply don't enjoy. There is no need for that. Enjoy walking and yoga.

Hatha Yoga

The goal of yoga is to balance the forces of the elements. The movement, or *asana,* of yoga creates strength, length, flexibility, comfort, and space in your body for your breath. The breath, or *pranayama,* of yoga lowers your blood pressure and that in turn calms the nervous energy and tension of the body and mind, thus relieving stress. The combination of asana and pranayama prepares the mind to receive meditation.

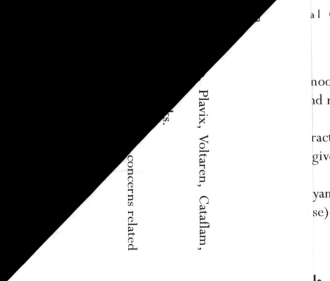

noon salutations.

...d moon energy of the body, representing the

...racticed in the West. What we commonly think ...given birth to power yoga, Bikram yoga, and

...yama (breathing), a short meditation or set-...se). You leave feeling grounded, at peace, and

Is

Yoga is for all people. Your physical situation does not prohibit you from practicing yoga. Yoga is designed to heal your perceived limitations.

Any of the following may be described as a physical situation, but I like to think of these situations as opportunities.

- Feeling old and having not worked out regularly. Yoga is an opportunity for me to age more gracefully, maintain balance, and sharpen my mind.
- Being inflexible and stiff. Yoga is an opportunity for me to lengthen and strengthen every major muscle group in my body. It will increase my stamina and balance.
- Being overweight. Yoga is an opportunity for me to move in an effortless way to facilitate weight loss. I will learn to modify my diet, how to eat more intentionally, and how to better enjoy my life.
- Being so overweight that a medical doctor would diagnose me as obese. Yoga is an opportunity for me to retake control of my health. Yoga is a way for me to slowly grow into my new physical and emotional form.
- Suffering from a medical condition. The yoga studio will take your medical conditions into consideration during practice. Any form of physical practice should be performed with the permission of your medical care provider.
- Suffering emotionally. The mental benefits of yoga are immeasurable. You will be given the tools to overcome your suffering and to see the world in a different light. Yoga heals.
- Not having time to attend a class or workshop. The goal of yoga instruction is to make you independent in your yoga practice. Once the initial investment of time is made in lessons, you will have the knowledge and experience to do yoga on your own, without an instructor.

I have personally taught yoga to people confined to wheelchairs and hospital beds, so I know that all people really can do yoga. During your Cleanse, your practice may be to relax on the floor and allow yourself to drift. This is called *Shavasana* or the "corpse" pose, and it is truly one of our most powerful poses.

Yoga and Religion

Yoga predates religion. Yoga is a spiritual practice that cultivates an understanding that divinity is expressed in our ordinary existence. When you attend a yoga class, you might hear theological or philosophic ideas, or none at all, depending upon the teacher and where you are practicing. Most health clubs eliminate all spiritual discussion, which turns yoga into a physical exercise only. I personally like to hear others' views of the world, and I go to yoga with an open mind and heart. When I teach, I pull out bits from all the great masters: Jesus, Buddha, Krishna, and more. There are powerful lessons to be gleaned from all religions.

The following discussion about yoga will be a nice read for your bedtime practice of reading something spiritual instead of watching television.

The Eight Limbs of Yoga

There are eight "limbs" or "branches" of yoga. The physical movement you currently identify as yoga is just one limb of the tree. The limbs, when practiced in concert, become part of your chemistry. They help you to live a good life and to find your life's purpose. They guide you to make better choices, cultivate better habits, and realize better relationships. They are only understood through the tangible experience of yoga; they cannot be intellectually understood. You must practice yoga for the understanding to unfold. After the Cleanse process, I encourage you to reread this section and comprehend it in a new way.

First Branch of Yoga: The Yamas, or Rules of Social Behavior

The *yamas* are rules of social conduct that engage you with others. They are important because we must have rules of conduct in each society that are clearly understood. Depending on where you live and your culture, your yamas will differ. Pantanjali, who codified yoga, broke the yamas down as follows:

Ahimsa (Nonviolence)

Ahimsa is the foundation for all that we do in yoga. It's the most important rule; if you only practice this one rule, the rest will follow. Ahimsa is the practice of not harming yourself, others, or your planet through violent thought, word, or deed. It is a caution to monitor your thoughts and always choose the more nourishing thought. Your thoughts become your words, your words become your deeds, and your deeds become your whole life. Begin with peaceful thoughts, and the rest will follow.

Satya (Truthfulness)

Satya is having integrity of thought, word, and deed. To be truthful, you must know your truth. Challenge yourself by asking, what do I believe?

Most people don't realize that the Buddha was a yogi. When speaking the truth, always begin with Ahimsa. Ask yourself the following Buddha questions before you speak:

Is it true?
Is it necessary?
Is it kind?
What would Buddha do?

Brachmacharya (Appropriate Use of One's Energy)

Brachmacharya has been very misunderstood in yoga because religion somehow made its way into Pantanjali's interpretation. Brachmacharya has been defined as "celibacy." It is my opinion that celibacy goes against our nature and is a religious construct. We are of nature, which is an expression of divinity, and therefore a healthy expression of sex is part of our experience.

Brachmacharya is the appropriate use of one's energies. By that, it is meant that sexuality should be enjoyed in a healthy and loving way. I personally believe that sex enjoyed in partnership with love is the most nourishing choice.

You can also think of Brachmacharya as how you spend your energy. Spending energy in un-fulfilling situations such as bad relationships, bad friendships, bad jobs, or gossiping can be very draining and unhealthy.

You can make this very simple by always asking yourself what is the most nourishing experience? Is it rock and roll or classical music playing in the background? Walking by a trash dumpster or walking in the middle of a field? Sex with someone you hardly know or sex with a partner who knows your body, your mind, and your heart?

Asteya (Honesty)

Asteya is translated as honesty, but you may ask, isn't honesty the same as truth (Satya)? Not exactly. Honesty is relinquishing the idea that things outside yourself will provide you happiness and security.

During the Cleanse we work on manifesting our hearts' desires. We then learn to simply release all of this as we begin to realize that we have all that we could ever desire already in this moment.

Aparigraha (Generosity)

Aparigraha is the shifting from ego responses to soul responses.

During the Cleanse, you will learn to resonate with the Sattvic or pure qualities of your soul. You will embrace and accept your ego because it is beautiful, and it is giving you your personality and your experience here in this realm as yourself, but you will learn to respond instead of react. You will bring the pure qualities of your soul into your responses, thereby diminishing the dramas of life that ego responses can create. You will learn to make heart-centered choices.

Second Branch of Yoga: Niyama, or Rules of Personal Behavior

How do you live when no one is watching? If you are living a balanced life, these characteristics will develop on their own.

Shoucha (Purity)

Shoucha is making choices that are nourishing to your body, mind, and soul. Always choose the more nourishing choice, including food, exercise, who to spend time with, what to listen to, and what to watch on TV. Choose your emotions and experiences.

Santosa (Present Moment Awareness)

Santosa translates to "present moment awareness" and "acceptance without resignation." Relinquish your attachment to the need for control, power, and approval.

When we practice present moment awareness, we accept things as they are. We accept that right now everything is perfect or, as it should be.

Tapas (Yoga as a Way of Living)

Tapas is the disciplined practice of yoga on and off your mat. During the Cleanse, you will learn a routine to live by that echoes or follows the rhythms of nature. Once you tap into those rhythms, tapas becomes easy.

Svadhyana (Turning Inward)

Svadhyaya means "looking inside." Your value comes from a deep connection with spirit. During the Cleanse, you will experience many spiritual exercises to take you deep into your psyche. You will explore why you think what you think, why you believe what you believe, and why you have thoughts.

Ishwara-Pranidhana (Letting Go)

This niyama is about surrendering to Spirit and having an attitude of devotion in all that you do. It is a tangible experience that cannot be intellectually understood. During the Cleanse, you will begin to foster a tangible relationship with Spirit.

"*Being in deep devotion comes as a surprise the first time, because it is so difficult for people to feel even love, and devotion is the highest form of love....If love is the flower, then devotion is just the fragrance. You cannot catch hold of it. You can feel it, you can smell it, you can be surrounded by it, you can be drowned in it, but you cannot catch hold of it. It is not that material.*" ~ Osho

What Do You Stand For?

I've added this niyama myself, and I think Pantanjali would approve of it. This niyama is a challenge for you to develop your own personal rule. What do you live for? What do you value? What defines you? Mother Teresa's personal niyama was to treat every person as she would Jesus coming off the cross. This allowed her to serve lepers and untouchables with loving kindness. Martin Luther King's personal niyama was to teach tolerance and the meaning of freedom to the world. Gandhi's personal niyama was peaceful resistance. Those are well-known names and ambitious goals. Your personal niyama need not be so grand. It can be simply to serve your family. Ask yourself, what is my niyama? Spend some time thinking about it.

Third Branch of Yoga: Asana, or Postures

Asana is the disciplined practice of yoga embodied by the poses most people recognize.

Fourth Branch of Yoga: Pranayama, or Prana, Life Force, Breathing

Pranayama is the disciplined practice of breathing. Breathe in. Breath out. Be aware that you are breathing. It's as simple as that.

Fifth Branch of Yoga: Pratyahara, or Tuning Into Your Subtle Sensory Experience

Pratyahara is the practice of becoming acutely aware of your senses to the point that you are able to withdraw your senses from the world. To practice, you focus on your senses and ultimately you are able to turn them off. This practice aids in meditation and in mindfulness.

You will learn how to pay attention to your five senses and recognize the ways in which your body reacts. Begin by spending time alone in silence.

Sixth Branch of Yoga: Dharana, or Mastery of Attention and Intention

Dharana, Dhyana, and Samdhi all have to do with meditation. They are practiced concurrently. Together, they make Samyama, or control.

Dharana is the point at which the mind needs an instrument to play in order to keep it from wandering. This instrument may be a mantra, japa mala, or even attention to breath. During the Cleanse, we use the mantra "so hum." Note that even the most experienced meditators have days when the mind wanders and they go back to an instrument. That is why Dharana, Dhyana, and Samdhi are practiced together and not consecutively.

Be aware of your intentions; pay attention to clues. Notice synchronicity.

Seventh Branch of Yoga: Dhyana, or Development of Witnessing Awareness

You are in this world, but not of this world. Your soul does not change, but everything else does.

Be aware of the silent presence that resides within you. As you experience the drama of living, remove yourself from it and watch it. Notice your thoughts and emotions as if you are watching a movie unfold.

Eighth Branch of Yoga: Samadhi, or the State of Being Settled in Pure, Unbounded Awareness

Know yourself as a spiritual being disguised as a human. Samadhi is not easily defined or described. It is a state of being known as bliss. This experience is unique to the practitioner. You will know when you have entered Samadhi without any definition or description coming from outside yourself. Samadhi is experienced at and in death, so we will all have this experience.

Enjoy the journey!

Spiritual Study

Pamela's Recommended Reading List

Spending time away from the frenzy of electronic media is critical to your success during the Cleanse. Reading works by inspirational authors or poets or spiritual texts is a calming replacement for the time we usually spend in front of the TV.

Remember that the stimuli you take in, especially before bedtime, are brought into your dreams. Let your dreams be a place for you to heal, process emotions, and resolve your own problems, not those of the world.

You'll notice that I love books. If you have a favorite, please share it with me. You are not required to read all of the books on this list, but I recommend reading at least some of them.

"There are only two ways to live your life. One is as though nothing is a miracle. The other is as though everything is a miracle."

~ ALBERT EINSTEIN

"We do not see things as they are. We see them as we are."

~ THE TALMUD

Eat, Taste, Heal: Ayurveda, by Thomas Yarema

Thomas Yarema writes about Ayurveda in a way that is simple and easy. I recommend starting here before undertaking deeper Ayurvedic studies. This book also includes delicious recipes.

Perfect Health, by Dr. Deepak Chopra

This describes the program I am certified to teach through the Chopra Center for Wellbeing. Dr. Chopra is an inspiration. Everything he writes is awesome.

Yoga & Ayurveda: Self-Healing and Self-Realization, by Dr. David Frawley

When you are ready to dive into the deep end of Ayurveda and yoga, this is the book for you.
The Seven Spiritual Laws of Yoga, by Dr. Deepak Chopra, Dr. David Simon, and Claire Diab
This is the other set of principles that I am certified to teach through the Chopra Center for Wellbeing. I love this book because it clearly outlines a daily practice that is simple and easy to follow. Each day is themed with a lesson, a mantra, and a chakra. It's simple and elegant.

True Love, by Thich Nat Hahn

Everything this Zen Buddhist Master writes inspires me. This is my favorite, though, because he describes an actual practice we can do in each moment with all the people in our lives to facilitate loving relationships. It's a little book that is simple to read.

Words I Wish I Wrote, by Robert Fulghum

This is the book that started me on my journey into yoga and Ayurveda. Robert Fulghum, who is most known for his book *Everything I Need to Know I Learned in Kindergarten,* wrote this book for charity. It is a collection of quotes and poems that most inspire him. After reading this book, I went on to read every single author he mentions in the book.

Conversations with God, by Neale Walsh

Walsh introduces concepts and ideas that you may have never considered. As always, I encourage you to listen to your heart in these matters. It might get you thinking in ways that help you find greater clarity about your own beliefs.

Codependent No More: How to Stop Controlling Others and Start Caring for Yourself, by Melody Beattie

Melody Beattie has been writing about emotional healing for thirty years. I recommend you peruse them all and pick the one that most resonates with you. As the adult child of an

alcoholic and abusive family, I have certainly ha
pendent issues. Sometimes it's helpful to read a
stereotypical patterns. During the Cleanse, you
makers" that are directing your life, with you un
this book.

Healing the Addictive Mind: Freeing Yourself from Ad
Jampols

If you've ever thought, "Wow, I may be addicte
is no judgment here, only understanding. Mr. Jamp
around the idea of addiction. It's a great place to g
falling into any stereotypical behavior patterns related to addiction.

Yoga of Heart: The Healing Power of Intimate Connection, by Mark Whitwell

Mark talks about the devotional nature of yoga and relates it to a time before religion. This book speaks to loving your ordinary life, but realizing that your life is extraordinary in every single way. I think this book will really help you to enjoy your journey.

Here are some others who may inspire you, in no particular order: Buddha, Confucius, Ralph Waldo Emerson, Mahatma Gandhi, Jesus, Martin Luther King, the Dalai Lama, Ramana Maharshi, Bob Marley, Muhammad, Pat Robertson, Rumi, Kahlil Gibran, Rabindranath Tagore, Hafiz, Cat Stevens, Mother Teresa, Lao Tzu, Malcolm X, Jerry Garcia, Albert Camus, Dylan Thomas, Franz Kafka, Marcel Proust, Beatrix Potter, Ranier Maria Rilke, Albert Einstein, Paramahansa Yogananda, David Hawkins, Sri Nisargadatta Maharaj, Pema Chodron, Carlos Casteneda, St. Francis of Assisi, Thomas Merton, Peace Pilgrim, Gary Zukav, Byron Katie, Tao Te Ching, Norman Vincent Peale, Richard Rose, Victor Frankl, William Blake, and Walt Whitman.

Journaling

Key components of The Elemental Cleanse are managing stress, tapping into creativity, and self-study, or what we call *svadyaya* in yoga. The perfect way to combine all of this is to establish a journal practice. Many people have great resistance to writing down their thoughts and emotions for fear that someone will read what they have written. If this is the case for you, purchase a password-protected computer program to use as your journal or simply store your journal in a private spot.

Your life is going to shift, not just during the next twenty-eight days, but over the next few years as your consciousness expands and you learn to connect more deeply with Spirit. I've had so many precious and amazing experiences and am grateful for the record of my experiences contained in my journals.

effective tool for managing and reducing stress. Simply by writing down
s and emotions, especially those related to anger, grief, and loneliness, you
to feel happier. Once you name the emotion, it starts to dissipate.
rch even points to a boost in the immunity system from journaling.
hile you are writing (a left-brain activity), your right brain (the dreamer) is allowed
space and time to free flow. This boosts your creativity.

Journaling enhances your ability to problem solve. Writing down your problems is a
concrete way to come up with multiple plans to resolve areas of conflict in your life. As
you write, you are able to step back and see the big picture, others' points of view, and
alternate solutions.

Journal every day. Begin by setting a timer for ten minutes and work up to twenty minutes
per day. Put your pen to paper and begin writing every thought you have. Keep your pen moving.
If you have to, simply write "nothing, nothing, nothing" until your next thought arises. I call this
type of journaling "Fire Pages," because you are getting the force of the Fire or Pitta out of your
head. Your journal does not have to make sense. Simply stream your consciousness from your
head to your journal. No one will see it and correct spelling does not matter. This is a helpful
practice if you have many thoughts during meditation that you cannot seem to slow.

You can also journal in a directed manner around the spiritual exercises that you will be
participating in during your Cleanse. Toward the end of the Cleanse, you will be writing your
life story. Begin to think about that now by asking yourself, what is my story? How do I want my
story to end?

For more inspiration and to boost your enthusiasm toward journaling, I recommend a book
called *Writing Down Your Soul,* by Janet Conner. Her personal story is inspirational, and she will
motivate you to write.

Modifications to the Cleanse

Many people undertaking the Cleanse are experiencing a challenging situation in their life, either physical or emotional in nature. The Cleanse is a way to reveal the root cause of the disease or challenging situation and to create a balanced mind and body.

Each person is unique; your experience of the Cleanse will be unique. You may need to modify the Cleanse slightly to meet your needs or address your situation. Please read the following sections as they pertain to you, but *everyone* should read the first section, which concerns healthy weight loss.

- What Is Healthy Weight Loss?
- I Do Not Need to Lose Weight
- Arthritis
- Diabetes
- Irritable Bowel Syndrome
- Pregnancy and Nursing
- Raw Foodies
- Depression, Anxiety, and Grief

What Is Healthy Weight Loss?

Health is not measured in pounds. Healthy weight loss is generally accepted to be around 1 to 2 pounds per week. Most participants in the Cleanse lose 6 to 12 pounds in twenty-eight days. I've had many lose 15 to 20 pounds. Usually, this happens with people who (1) get super-excited to Cleanse and either start early or extend the third or the final week, thereby extending the duration of the Cleanse; (2) give up their less-favorable habits more rapidly and do not pick them back up; or (3) need to lose in excess of forty pounds.

Weight gain is an Earth (Kapha) imbalance. When you think of the Earth, think about something that is heavy, dense, stable, and inert. If you have added Earth and these properties to your body, then you need to understand that it's going to take some effort to get the Earth moving. Earth moves very slowly. Remember that you didn't go to bed one night and wake up overweight the next morning. It took time to put that extra Earth on your body, and it's going to take time to take it off. Be patient with yourself.

Earth is a powerful energy. Once is gets moving, it has stamina. During the first week of the Cleanse, most participants will experience a diminishing of bloating and their clothes will begin to fit better. The second week of the Cleanse begins the weight loss. Week 3 and Week 4 offer significant shifting in Kapha and therefore excess weight.

The extra effort through exercise to get Kapha moving can be achieved through a gentle yoga practice and daily walking. In fact, if you are currently in any fitness routine that brings you a sense of suffering (running, biking, swimming, lifting weights), I ask that you set those routines aside. For the month of the Cleanse, I want you to experience nourishing and pleasurable exercise. Of course, if you realize a state of total Zen while doing any of your exercises and you love them, then stay with them in addition to the yoga you do.

Set realistic goals for yourself, taking into account healthy weight loss. You can count on losing the first 6 to 12 pounds over the next twenty-eight days. After that, plan to lose 1 to 2 pounds per week. You will do this by sticking with the eating plan for your element.

One of the best aspects about the Cleanse is that it teaches you to love yourself at whatever weight you are. You will learn to free yourself from the attachment to the ideal that you are supposed to look a certain way. The bottom line is that you are supposed to *feel* a certain way: vibrant, joyous, and energetic. The excess weight will come off as a side effect to coming back to balance.

Key Factors for Losing Weight During the Cleanse

- Daily movement
- Daily rest (meditation)
- Stress reduction
- Elimination of less-favorable habits
- Including beans, veggies, grains, and fruits (in that proportionate order) in meals. Maximize beans and minimize grains.
- Daily routine
- Healthy serving size
- Elimination of snacking

Weight Gain and Stress

Stress causes weight gain. During periods of stress the forces of The Wind and The Fire go out of balance, in that order. These are forces that move or transform. These are high-energy forces that are aggravating when they are out of balance. Our mind and our body naturally know that we need to be grounded and that we can achieve that feeling with food. We reach for quick, easy, sweet and starchy foods to try to get back into balance. These foods also give us the emotional high of feeling the love. It's natural, instinctive, and healthy to reach for grounding foods in time of stress. Unfortunately, we live a life where the stress never ends and we are constantly reaching out for that sweet taste.

It is critical to manage your stress levels if you want to shift the element of The Earth off your body. It's hard to imagine that sitting still and meditating is going to help you lose weight, but it will.

I Do Not Need to Lose Weight

Most of us have the perception that if someone appears thin and in good shape, they must be in good health. What we can't see are the potentially toxic thoughts and buildup of *ama*, or toxicity, in their veins and organs. Many participants in the Cleanse do not need to lose weight. They come for a myriad of other reasons including the desire to do the following:

- Recover from disease
- Eliminate ama from body and mind
- Establish a meditation practice
- Establish a yoga practice
- Connect to Spirit
- •Transform their jobs, relationships, or family

The Cleanse is designed to "uplift" the body and mind. If you do not need to lose weight but you follow the eating plan, you will lose weight. To maintain your weight, adhere to the following modifications:

- Add five additional minutes to your daily meditation practice.
- Practice gentle, beginners, yin, or slow vinyasa flow yoga.
- Stay warm. When walking outside in the cold, cover your throat and head.
- Seek out heat therapy. If you have access to a hot tub, sauna, or steam room, use it regularly during the Cleanse.
- Follow the eating routine. That means three meals each day around the same time each day. Planning is critical, as well as shopping and cooking. Many Cleansers who do not need to lose weight have a Wind body and a Wind mind. They have a hard time planning and sticking to a routine. It is essential that you prioritize food this month.
- You may eat more than two cups of food at any given meal. Eat until you begin to feel full.
- You may snack, but wait two hours between snacking and eating a meal. The Yogi Breakfast is a perfect snack food and a perfect way to start your day if you find breakfast to be a challenge due to lack of routine or morning appetite. The recipe can be found at the back of the book, under Supplemental Information.
- Portion your food on your plate in the following order:

1. Whole grains including pasta
2. Vegetables
3. Beans (mostly legumes)
4. Fruits
5. Nuts, seeds, and oils

A meal is about two cups of food. The largest portion of your meal is whole grains. The next largest is vegetables, and so on. You are favoring whole grains and vegetables over all other food.

Consume four to eight teaspoons of oil each day. You may ingest flaxseed oil or cook with sesame, olive, or another oil of your choice.

If you are the Wind body type, you may continue to consume organic meat (poultry, fish, and eggs) up to five times each week until the final week of the Cleanse. The final week (fourth week) will be your only non-meat week.

Arthritis and The Elemental Cleanse

Arthritis affects 40 percent of Americans between the ages of forty-five and sixty-five and up to 60 percent of Americans over the age of sixty-five. There are more than one hundred different types of arthritis affecting more than 70 million people.

Ayurveda considers arthritis to be a disease resulting from aggravation of The Wind (Vata) dosha, which results in an accumulation of ama or toxins as The Earth (Kapha) is pushed out of balance. This accumulation is the result of long-term, improper digestion or weak digestive fire (agni).

The cure for arthritis is to rid the body of the accumulated toxins. This is exactly what we do during The Elemental Cleanse. If you are suffering from arthritis, I suggest the following:

- Rid your diet of meat and dairy during the first week. You will not suffer any withdrawal from these two habits, so it is fine to do in one week. It will make a huge difference in how quickly your agni increases. Favor beans, veggies, whole grains, and fruits (in that proportionate order).
- During the Cleanse, I explain that your initial personal yoga practice can simply be to lie in Shavasana or corpse pose for ten minutes each day. This practice is also good for you, but prop your legs straight up against a wall for Shavasana to boost your immune system. Your yoga practice should include more movement as well. Plan to attend gentle yoga three times a week.
- Ginger, neem, and guggulu are the recommended herbal therapy. Consider doubling your intake of all three. That means taking two tablets in the morning and two tablets at night of neem and guggulu.
- Heat your sesame oil in a pan or in an oil warmer prior to your self-administered massages. Do this morning and night, and place special emphasis on working the oil deeply into your achy joints. Add cinnamon to the sesame oil.
- Seek out hot therapy such as steam rooms, saunas, and hot tubs. If you do not have access to any of these, soak in a hot bath.

Arthritis and the Doshas

Arthritis is a chronic condition that will improve dramatically as a result of the Cleanse. Post-Cleanse, consider what type of arthritis you are experiencing and follow the routine for that body type.

The Wind: Popping and cracking of the joints characterizes arthritis resulting from a Wind imbalance.

The Fire: Arthritis that is the result of a Fire imbalance is characterized by inflammation and pain. The joints are swollen, red, and possibly even hot to the touch. Moving aggravates the pain.

The Earth: Joints that are stiff and swollen characterize arthritis that is a result of an Earth imbalance. They may feel cold and clammy to the touch. Moving the joints tends to relieve the pain.

Many Cleansers who suffer from arthritis continue their herbal therapy after the twenty-eight-day Cleanse program.

Diabetes and The Elemental Cleanse

Roughly 26 million people in the United States suffer from diabetes. Another 76 million people are termed "prediabetic." In 2007, it was estimated that $174 billion dollars were spent on diabetes. Prediabetes is reversible with routine and nutrition. It is unclear if type 2 diabetes is reversible in this way, and type 1 diabetes is not reversible, but you can manage it, and you can have a better quality of life, by making sensible changes to your routine and diet.

The following information is from the American Diabetes Association:

Type 1 diabetes is usually diagnosed in children and young adults, and was previously known as juvenile diabetes. In type 1 diabetes, the body does not produce insulin. Insulin is a hormone needed to convert sugar, starches and other food into energy. Only 5% of people with diabetes have this form of the disease. With the help of insulin therapy and other treatments, even young children with type 1 diabetes can learn to manage their condition and live long, healthy, happy lives.

Type 2 diabetes is the most common form of diabetes. In type 2 diabetes, either the body does not produce enough insulin or the cells ignore the insulin. Insulin is necessary for the body to use glucose for energy. When you eat food, the body breaks down all of the sugars and starches into glucose, which is the basic fuel for the cells. Insulin takes the sugar from the blood into the cells. When glucose builds up in the blood instead of going into cells, it can lead to diabetes complications.

Diabetes in Ayurveda is generally considered an Earth or Kapha disorder, although an Ayurvedic physician has up to twenty-four classifications for diabetes. It results from a weak digestive fire or agni. The first step to reducing and/or reversing the effects of diabetes is to cleanse the body and mind of accumulated toxins. The Elemental Cleanse is the perfect course to learn to manage and mitigate the effects of diabetes.

Why the Cleanse Works for Diabetes

The Elemental Cleanse will assist you in learning how to eat a healthy diet. The Cleanse will slowly take you off of your typical "American" diet and teach you to incorporate healthy foods and ways of eating for managing diabetes.

During the Cleanse, we focus on eating foods with a low glycemic index (GI). Plus, you will learn how to favor foods that are all part of a healthy diabetic diet. These foods are:

- Beans and legumes
- Leafy greens and vegetables
- Whole grains that are unprocessed
- Fruits

We eliminate meats and most saturated fat. We learn to cook with oils that are high in good fats. We eliminate dairy that is high in calories and saturated fat. We eliminate sugar beverages and learn to favor water and tea. We learn about portion control to facilitate weight loss. We avoid starchy vegetables of little value such as white potatoes.

Things to Know While Cleansing

You should cleanse with the approval of your physician. You should invest in vegetarian cookbooks that specifically address the management of diabetes. If you are taking the time to learn about a vegetarian or vegan lifestyle, you might as well incorporate an education about your disease.

You may have a snack. We embrace healthy snacking. The recommendation for the Cleanse is to eat three meals per day equal to 1.5 to 2 cups each meal. You may find that you need to eat six meals per day, or three meals with snacks. You may simply need to eat more to adjust your insulin needs. The first three weeks of the Cleanse should be spent slowly making the adjustments.

The eating routine includes eating around the same time each day. This will help you to manage your blood sugar level. Your meals will be well planned and well balanced to include beans, grains, vegetables, and fruits. The starchier food groups will only account for one-fourth of your plate.

The closer a food is to nature, the lower the GI. That means to choose unprocessed and whole foods. Eliminating the color white from your diet is an easy way to eliminate many processed foods. Processed sugar, flour, and grains, including bread that is white, are processed. Whole foods include vegetables and fruits that are fresh as well as whole grains like rice, barley, and quinoa.

Beans

- Dried beans such as black, lima, and pinto
- Lentils, mung, dal, and dahl (*dal* is the Sanskrit word for "lentil")
- Split peas and black-eyed peas

Nonstarchy Vegetables

- Alfalfa sprouts
- Amaranth
- Artichoke
- Artichoke hearts
- Asparagus
- Bamboo shoots
- Beans: green, Italian, yellow, or wax
- Bean sprouts
- Broccoli
- Brussels sprouts
- Cabbage
- Carrots
- Cauliflower
- Celery
- Chicory
- Chinese cabbage
- Cucumber
- Eggplant
- Green onions or scallions
- Greens: beet, collard, dandelion, kale, mustard, or turnip
- Jicama
- Kohlrabi
- Leeks
- Lettuce: endive, escarole, leafy varieties, Romaine, or iceberg
- Mixed vegetables without corn, peas, or pasta
- Mushrooms
- Okra
- Onions
- Parsley
- Peppers (all varieties)
- Radishes
- Rutabaga
- Sauerkraut
- Snow peas or pea pods
- Spinach
- Summer squash
- Swiss chard
- Tomato, raw
- Tomato juice (low sodium)
- Tomato paste (low sodium)
- Tomato sauce (low sodium)

- Turnips
- Vegetable juice cocktail (low sodium)
- Water chestnuts
- Watercress
- Zucchini

Fruits

With the exception of watermelon and pineapple, fruits have a low GI.

Exercise

Regular walking and yoga will help your body regulate your blood sugar level.

Meditation

Meditation helps you reduce your levels of stress hormones. This can keep your blood sugar and blood pressure under control, with the additional benefit of a reduction in the risk of heart disease.

Herbal Therapy

Neem is approved by the Indian government and is sold by the pharmaceutical industry in India as a treatment for diabetes. While studies have not been performed in the United States, the studies in India show a reduction in insulin requirements.

Guggul is used in India to treat obesity, decrease high cholesterol, and manage weight gain. Many of these same issues affect diabetics. Some researchers are advocating the use of guggul to specifically treat diabetes although studies have not yet been performed in the United States.

Triphala is an antioxidant and is believed to positively affect the pancreas. No conclusive studies have been performed.

Many Cleansers who suffer from diabetes continue their herbal therapy after the twenty-eight-day Cleanse process.

Irritable Bowel Syndrome (IBS)

Many Cleansers suffer from IBS. It is believed that one in six people suffer from IBS, and most of the sufferers are women. IBS can be debilitating.

Abdominal cramping and pain as well as unpredictability in bowel movements characterize irritable bowel syndrome. There is no known cause of IBS, although it is thought that it stems from an infection.

Stress is definitely linked with IBS. Your digestive system responds to emotion. In fact, your colon and your brain are deeply connected through your autonomic nervous system. I've always found it fascinating that the intestines have a brain-like appearance. For me, that is a good reminder that my digestive tract and brain are linked.

If you are suffering from IBS, the Cleanse is going to help you dramatically. First, it is going to help you manage and minimize your stress levels. Second, it is going to teach you to eat a pure, or *sattvic,* diet. You should do the following things in addition to what is recommended during the Cleanse.

- Cook all of your food.
- Add raw honey to your diet. You can put it in your tea if you choose.
- Drink a lassi each day. Lassis do contain yogurt (dairy) so you get a pass on totally eliminating dairy. Buy high-quality, organic yogurt. The recipe is found in the Supplemental Information section at the end of the book.
- Add lemon to your ginger tea.
- Drink a full glass of room temperature water as soon as you awaken each morning. Keep the glass of water by your bed and drink before your feet even hit the floor. This is part of the Daily Routine, but lots of folks overlook this. Don't overlook it.
- Go directly to the bathroom each morning and sit with the intention to eliminate. You may or may not eliminate, but you are establishing a routine for elimination that your body will embrace.
- As long as you are not suffering withdrawal, eliminate caffeine over the course of two, not three weeks. We will discuss caffeine further later in the book. You should intend to permanently eliminate caffeine.
- Add the following herbal therapy:
  1. Flaxseed oil, 2 to 6 capsules per day
  2. Daily probiotic
  3. Shatavari
  4. Aloe vera juice (you can add this to your Lassi)

Pregnancy, Nursing, and The Elemental Cleanse

Many pregnant and nursing mothers have participated in the Cleanse. It's a meaningful undertaking for those who want to learn to nourish their babies in the most holistic way. For nursing mothers, it can be a bit more challenging, simply because the baby must be your priority and your sleep is disrupted. The Cleanse can teach the nursing mother to make good choices for herself and her family, and to prioritize so that she can effectively take care of her family. Whether you are pregnant or nursing, please be sure to check with your doctor before beginning.

Modifications for Cleansing

Do not take neem or triphala guggulu. Simply set those aside to be taken at a later date when you are no longer pregnant or nursing.

You may take triphala. Triphala will help to facilitate elimination as it acts as a mild laxative. It is a blend of three fruits and is perfectly safe for mothers. You can purchase triphala at www. elementalom.com.

Add flaxseed oil to your diet in capsule or liquid form, and use iodized organic salt when cooking.

Eat more. The Cleanse eating routine suggests three meals each day. Each meal consists of 1.5 to 2 cups of food. However, you will need to eat more than this and add snacks as well. Your calorie requirements will increase by about 300 calories per day during your second trimester. Nursing mothers should watch their milk supply. If it is low, you may not be consuming enough calories.

Protein. You will need more protein than women who are not pregnant and not nursing. Most people on average only need around 49 grams of protein a day. You will need around 70 grams. Look to non-animal sources of protein such as lentils, sesame seeds, peanuts, almonds, tofu, soymilk, and whole grains. The yogi drink recommended during the Cleanse will be a suitable (and delicious) snack for you.

Meat as a source of protein. Follow your cravings. If you feel that you must continue to consume three to five servings of organic meat each week, please choose eggs or fish over all other meats. Do not eat red meat, including pork.

Calcium. You need more calcium. Continue to take your supplements daily and look to add calcium-rich foods to your diet, such as fortified soymilk, quinoa, beans, kelp, sesame seeds, figs, and fortified orange juice. Some herbs, such as basil, cinnamon, and thyme, contain up to 80 grams of calcium each.

Prenatal vitamin. Your prenatal vitamin should include an iron supplement along with all the other supplements needed for pregnancy. I would suggest you continue to take this while nursing. Talk to your physician about a prescription-strength vitamin. Nursing mothers do not need as much iron as pregnant mothers.

Modify yoga for pregnancy. Find a studio that offers prenatal classes. During the first trimester, it is not usually necessary to modify the poses, but you may find that a gentle and nourishing class helps you to maintain energy and balance. During the second trimester, you must start modifying your practice to accommodate your pregnancy.

Meditation. Many yogis experience a deep bonding with their developing babies during pregnancy. If you are nursing, you can bring mantra into those 3:00 a.m. feedings gently rocking, feeding and reciting your mantra. The calmer you become, the calmer your little one will become.

Raw Foods Diet and The Elemental Cleanse

Many people are advocates for raw food diets and have a positive experience with them. Ayurveda does hold a place for the unique constitution that can thrive on a raw food diet. This would be a person who is a Fire (Pitta) body type or some balance of Fire/Earth (Pitta/Kapha). This type of person has naturally strong digestion and more heat. I believe that this person also needs a very strong presence of Fire in the mind, as it takes incredible planning and discipline to maintain a raw foods diet and appropriately meet all of your nutritional needs.

If you are choosing this raw food lifestyle and you feel great, that's awesome! If you are suffering physically or emotionally from any of the following, ask yourself if you are getting enough energy of the Earth or Kapha in your life to ground the uplifting nature of your diet.

- Lack of vitality
- Always cold
- Weak digestive digestion
- Cravings
- Stalled weight loss due to low metabolism
- Emaciation
- Amenorrhea (menstrual cycles cease), even in young women
- Loss of libido
- Hair loss and nail problems
- Dental erosion
- Insomnia and neurological problems
- Constipation
- Diarrhea
- Infertility

If you find that you are suffering from any of these or if you are participating in The Elemental Cleanse and do not wish to participate in cooked food, you will need to make the following modifications to the Cleanse:

- Daily meditation of no less than twenty minutes.
- Self-oil massage with sesame oil (it's heating externally and internally). Heat your oil prior to your massage.
- Vigorous yoga or exercise producing sweat with an extended rest (Shavasana) of no less than ten minutes to ground your energy afterward.
- Spice up your food with pungent spices like pepper and cayenne.
- Eat your food at room temperature.
- Take a daily dose of triphala (Ayurvedic blend of three fruits promoting digestion and elimination).
- Drink hot teas (ginger tea is the best). Add citrus (lemon or lime) to your teas.
- Add fruit juices and vegetable juices to your diet.
- Use a food processor or blender to pre-digest the food you consume.
- Take a daily dose of flaxseed oil. You may consume up to 6 to 8 teaspoons of oil each day for healthy digestion.
- Use ginger elixir before each meal to stoke your digestive fire. The elixir consists of grated ginger marinated in sea salt and lemon. Take a pinch before each meal.
- Go for a ten-minute walk after you eat.

- Seek out heat therapy; dress warmly, covering the throat and head; use saunas, hot baths, hot tubs, hot yoga (if appropriately acclimated and not more than twice a week), and sun.
- Go to bed by 10:00 p.m. and arise by 6:00 a.m.

The final week of The Elemental Cleanse is modified for those on a raw food diet. Food will be blended and processed and, without exception, at room temperature. Focus will be on vegetables over fruits. The final week may be shortened to just three days.

I find that people who take the Cleanse and are raw foodies are not taking the Cleanse to clean out their bodies. Most are interested in what Ayurveda has to offer and are curious about the spiritual aspects of the Cleanse. Great benefit can be received through the emotional, mental, and spiritual Cleansing process. Shift your focus to journaling, meditation, walking, and yoga. Because you already have a healthy diet, the food portion will be easy for you and not a focus.

Most of the raw foodies I know are very attached to their diet because they have put a lot of effort into this lifestyle and they have seen benefits. That's perfect! Simply be aware of the imbalance that a raw food diet can potentially cause if not balanced with the emotional and physical body. You will simply have to focus more on grounding your energy through meditation, yoga, and warmth. Raw food creates high prana. This always sounds good, as we perceive prana to be a positive force. Prana, however, is a neutral force. It goes where your mind goes. If you are happy, it increases the happy. If you are sad, destructive, critical, judgmental, or angry, it will also increase those. Too much prana, ungrounded, causes imbalance.

Depression, Anxiety, and Grief and The Elemental Cleanse

Modifications

The fact that you made the choice to participate in The Elemental Cleanse is a powerful sign that your situation is already starting to shift. I personally have suffered from depression and grief, and I know how hard it is to begin the process of coming up for air. Depending where you are in your process of healing from depression, anxiety, or grief, you may need to modify the Cleanse in the following ways.

If you find it difficult to sit with your eyes closed for meditation, please practice by simply opening your eyes a very tiny amount and take your focus to the floor in front of you or just beyond the tip of your nose. Some people benefit from staring at a candle flame or a picture. This will allow the "light of the world" to shine inward.

I want you to sit with your depression, grief, or anxiety. In the moment of intense emotion, remove yourself from your current situation and surroundings and go sit quietly. Take your attention to your breath and simply take long slow breaths in and out. Allow for the emotion to shift organically and observe the process. Do not detach from the emotion. Simply observe and honor it.

Uncomfortable emotions are based in fear. Fear turns to anger. Anger turns to grief. Grief turns to sadness. Sadness turns to forgiveness, and forgiveness turns to compassion. You are simply stuck somewhere in that loop during your intense experience. Cultivate awareness and watch your mind as an observer with a clinical eye. Educate your brain that all emotions evolve to compassion.

The meditation will actually increase your emotions before your mind calms. This is normal and natural. Notice this; journal your triggers and allow yourself the opportunity to shift your emotions up the scale. Do spend time each day in Shavasana (relaxation pose lying on your back) and allow for plenty of rest this month. Keep your activities to a minimum.

Find a simple affirmation to use daily instead of thinking random thoughts. This works to create a new loop or pattern in your brain. Some good affirmations are: *I am healing, I am happy, I am free, I am present,* and *I am accepting of all situations.* Throughout your day, as you notice you are having random thoughts, simply choose to think of these positive affirmations instead.

Become deeply attached to the process of journaling. It is an excellent way to get all of your thoughts and feelings out. You are going to experience a dynamic shift this month, and you may need personal attention as your emotions evolve. Reach out. It is also beneficial to work one on one with a counselor during this process.

Mostly, be kind to yourself. Treat yourself as you would a child experiencing this situation. Hold yourself, allow for the emotions, and give yourself time to feel all that you need to feel. Our society does not give us enough time or space to heal. Take this month to go through your process in a focused and clear manner.

If your situation is interfering with sleep, please purchase the book *Yoga Nidra* by Dr. Richard Miller. Use the CD at night to go to sleep. An herbal sleep aid I recommend is Valerian. It does cause drowsiness, so be sure to only take it at bedtime. Other supplements that that help include Ashwagandha and flaxseed oil.

Week 1 Overview

Let's Get Started!

Welcome to the beginning of your transformation! Week 1 is the Getting Organized Week. The focus is on establishing a meditation practice, organizing your schedule and pantry, and beginning to eliminate the less-favorable habits that are interfering with digestion.

Hopefully you have spent some time prior to this week reading about the Cleanse, taking the quizzes, finding a local yoga studio, and ordering your Cleansing Kit. If your kit has not arrived or if you have jumped right in without it, that's fine. You can begin your herbal therapy at any point.

The most important focus of Week 1 is to establish your meditation practice. I can't stress this enough. Meditation is critical to your success. Use the meditation scheduling sheet located in this chapter and in the back of the book to schedule each of your four weeks of the Cleanse. First, fill in the things that you *must* do in one color. This should include work, kids, and other necessities. Next, sit down with the yoga class schedule from the studio you chose and pick two to five yoga classes to attend each week. Finally, schedule ten minutes each day this first week to meditate. We will talk more about meditation in a bit.

Review the routines for eating, sleeping, and living. You will need to prepare. Explore recipes you wish to make, shop for groceries, and cook. Recipes are offered in the back of the book as well as on my website, www.elementalom.com. When you first look at the routines, you may become overwhelmed. Please trust that much of the routine does not take additional time; in fact, things like driving in silence, reading instead of watching TV, and planning your meals *save* time.

Set your intention to slowly eliminate your less-favorable habits. Many Cleansers get excited and eliminate everything immediately. This can cause you a lot of needless suffering and is *not* necessary. Habits like alcohol, sugar, caffeine, and processed food have a physically addictive nature. Your body will suffer if you do not slowly eliminate these items over the course of the Cleanse. Intend to follow my instructions for elimination.

Your spiritual exercise, or OM Work, for Week 1 is called, "The Good, the Bad, and the Ugly." The purpose of this exercise is to release your mind from thoughts of the past and to cultivate compassion and forgiveness for self and others. Intend to work on this. I've been teaching this

Cleanse for many years, and I consistently see people put their emotional healing work on the back burner. Once Cleansers are in Week 3, they realize that they should have been taking it more seriously and experience regret. Intend to do your work. This Cleanse works on all levels of existence, and I can't stress enough how important the spiritual work is.

Finally, enjoy the journey!

"It is better to enjoy the journey than to arrive."

~ Buddhist Proverb

Week I at a Glance

For Your Body

Eliminate one-third of your "less-favorable" habits. We will go over these in detail later in this section. That's one-third only! Please follow this or you will suffer withdrawal symptoms.

Eliminate red meat entirely from your diet. This includes beef and pork. You can still eat poultry and fish in moderation. I challenge you not to consume more than three to five servings a week.

Follow the Eating Routine

- Eat one vegetarian meal per day. Breakfast is the easiest to make vegetarian.
- Drink ginger tea. Sip it throughout your day. Use fresh ginger.
- Eliminate iced beverages from your diet. Sip room temperature water instead.
- Begin herbal therapy.
- Begin daily self-massage with sesame oil.
- Begin moving daily. Do yoga and walk thirty minutes each day.

For Your Mind

- Daily meditation of ten minutes.
- Create a sacred space for your meditation practice.
- Discuss your needs with your family. Ask them to support you.
- Clear your schedule for the next twenty-eight days. Remember, *no* is your most-used word this month.

For Your Spirit

- Daily silence. Drive in silence, cook in silence, and get ready for work in the morning in silence. Experience one hour of no talking each day.

- Spend some time in nature daily. This can be your thirty-minute walk.
- Create a positive affirmation for the week. Examples: I am healing, I am strong, my best is good enough.
- Complete your OM Work: "The Good, the Bad, and the Ugly."
- Journal every day.

Other

- Begin to read vegetarian recipes and explore the organic section of your grocery store.
- Clean out your pantry. Get rid of old spices, empty-calorie foods, and temptations.
- Begin to replace personal care and cleaning products with organic, good-for-the-planet products. Use what you have, but replace them with better choices as you run out.

Eliminating Your Less-Favorable Habits

Caffeine

Ahhhhh, the delicious smell of coffee in the morning. Believe me, I know. Each day I make French Press coffee. It's a ritual. I confess that I don't even make the best cup of coffee, but I love the process of boiling the water, stirring the grounds, and smelling that oh-so-delicious smell. I even love the sound the coffee makes when it splashes into my cup. On a normal day (by that I mean when I am not Cleansing) I have a cup of coffee. It's easy for me to not drink more because (1) I make bad coffee, and (2) I'm a Windy mind and usually forget where I've set my cup down after I've poured.

Most people, however, don't really know how much coffee they are drinking. The normal cup of today equals two of our normal cups of twenty years ago. Not to mention the "pick me ups" at the local coffee house, which seem like special treats but somehow turn into daily doses. And then there are soft drinks. On an average day, you could have two to four caffeinated beverages and not even realize it. Caffeine is highly addictive and really does sneak up on you.

Why We Eliminate Caffeine

Disease stems from poor digestion. Caffeine diminishes digestion. It puts out the fire, or agni, that we are working so hard to build. Caffeine dehydrates you. Drinking caffeine stresses the physical, mental, and emotional bodies. It increases the levels of glucocorticoids, such as cortisol, which actually make you hold onto fat. These are stress hormones.

Caffeine has a negative effect on the immune system, making it harder for your body to fight viral and bacterial infections. Caffeine causes your body to take oxygen from your brain to your extremities, causing memory loss. If you are drinking unfiltered coffee, you are increasing your LDL.

Caffeine and Your Body

Did you know that caffeine has a half-life of six hours in your body? That means that if you drink a coffee at 3:00 p.m., your body will have processed only half of it by 9:00 pm. This is disruptive to your sleep.

Caffeine is also quite addictive. When you stop using caffeine, you may experience symptoms of withdrawal in as few as twelve hours. Symptoms of withdrawal may include the following:

- Headaches
- Flu-like symptoms
- Irritability and restlessness
- Difficulty concentrating
- Muscle stiffness
- Chills
- Hot flashes
- Jitters
- Insomnia
- Anxiety
- Nausea
- Irregular heartbeat
- Flushed face

The good news is that caffeine is an addiction that is easy to break, and it doesn't have to be painful. Simply take the following steps to eliminate caffeine from your diet.

- Week 1: Go about your daily routine. When you get up in the morning and want your cup of coffee (or soda or tea), go ahead and make it just like you always do. Go to the sink and pour one-third off, then drink and enjoy. If you make a pot in the morning, go ahead and make the pot. Go to the sink and poor one-third off. Drink as usual. The same is true for sodas. Get your soda, pour one-third off, drink, and enjoy.
- Week 2: The same as above, but now you are pouring two-thirds of the cup away. This is the week when you may consider adding a decaf hot tea to your routine on top of the one-third-cup of coffee.
- Week 3: No more caffeine. Substitute decaffeinated teas and hot water with ginger instead.

During this process, if you suffer from any of the previously mentioned withdrawal symptoms, have a very small serving of caffeine to ease your suffering. A quarter cup of coffee will do the trick.

Most people are surprised that they are completely off caffeine by Week 2!

If you simply can't stand to hold a half-empty mug, substitute the coffee elimination with Yogi Breakfast. You will find the non-milk milk to be very filling.

Many Cleansers ask if they can simply switch from regular coffee to decaf coffee during their Cleanse. The answer is always no. While decaf coffee does contain trace amounts of caffeine, it is only around 1 to 5 mg. That is not a lot, so you might think, why not? The reason is that the point of the Cleanse is to learn new behaviors. To learn to drink teas infused with healing herbs or heated nondairy milks that are full of nutrition is a powerful lifestyle change that will benefit you in the long run.

The following table lists the caffeine content in some popular beverages. There is no recommended daily allowance for caffeine.

Brewed Coffee at home (8 oz.): 100 mg
Starbucks (12 oz.): 260 mg
Caribou Coffee (12 oz.): 230 mg
Dunkin Donuts coffee (10 oz.): 165 mg
Instant Coffee (8 oz.): 70 mg
Double espresso (2 oz.): 45–100 mg
Soda: 45–60 mg
Tea: 35–70 mg
Dark Chocolate: 25 mg
Red Bull: 80 mg
Bottled Yerba Matte Beverage (16 oz.): 140 mg
Diet Coke: 47 mg
Mountain Dew: 54 mg
Rockstar: 80 mg

Water and Ginger Tea

For purposes of the Cleanse, you need to know how to drink for your body type. The Wind (Vata) body should be more conscious about drinking water. Because of The Wind's dryness and lack of routine, more water is necessary, and focused drinking is also necessary. The rule of eight glasses of water a day applies to The Wind, unless you start to bloat.

The Fire (Pitta) body tends to run hot. The Fire type drinks when thirsty and does a great job of self-monitoring.

The Earth (Kapha) body has a lot of water in it already. Drink when you are thirsty, but don't attach to the idea that you are doing a Cleanse and need to flush your system. If you drink too much water, you will quickly bloat and completely put out your digestive fire. Four to eight glasses of water each day, depending on your thirst levels, is appropriate for The Earth. *Note:* For all body types, ginger tea consumption counts as water.

Please remember to drink your water at *room temperature*. Iced beverages put out your digestive fire, or agni. Also, *do not drink when you are eating.* Eat your food, wait, and then drink room temperature water if you are still thirsty.

Ginger Tea as Your Secret Weapon

Most days of my life, you will see me walking around with an insulated mug. In my mug is one of my cleansing secrets: ginger tea. I make my own by simply boiling water and pouring it over some freshly grated ginger. When I get bored, I add some lemon or a tea bag of some other flavor. I find that the ginger tea keeps my digestive fire high. It soothes me when my tummy hurts, and it is very effective at soothing the cramps I get with my menstrual cycle. Every sip is also a wonderful reminder to me to make good choices and to nourish my digestive fire.

For the purposes of Cleansing, I want you to drink two to four cups of ginger tea each day. You should purchase an insulated mug and a large root of ginger. Ginger root can be found in the produce section of the grocery store, usually by the mushrooms. One large root stored in a sealed plastic bag will last for the duration of the Cleanse.

Slice off about one inch of peeled ginger. You may simply put the whole chunk in the bottom of your mug or you may wish to slice or grate it. If you are grating it, you will be consuming more ginger. I will warn you that it is spicy; know your tolerance for spice.

Pour hot water over the ginger and plan to sip it all day. When the liquid is gone, you can usually add more water to the cube that is already in the bottom of the mug. It gets a little weaker as time goes by, but is usually good for about two to three servings.

When you begin the practice of drinking ginger tea, you will notice that you become very thirsty and that you are urinating frequently. This only lasts for two to three days, and then your body will be done with that initial flush of toxins.

Ginger simply makes everything better. You can hardly find an herbal holistic cure coming out of India that doesn't have some ginger in it. Ginger is thought to enhance other herbs and bring out their healing properties. In Ayurveda, ginger is deemed *sattvic,* which means that it is pure. It is used to tame The Wind in your body, invigorate The Earth, and stoke The Fire! It's heating, and it's wonderful for digestion.

Ginger is commonly used in Ayurveda for the following situations:

- Cold and flu
- Indigestion
- Vomiting
- Burping
- Gas and bloating
- Indigestion
- Menstrual cramping
- Arthritis
- Heart disease
- Headaches
- Hemorrhoids
- Diarrhea
- Asthma
- Bronchitis
- Depression

- Mental stress
- Exhaustion
- Restlessness and anxiety

Ginger is commonly used to treat nausea and vomiting, not only in day-to-day life, but also in patients being treated with chemotherapy. Researchers from the University of Michigan Comprehensive Cancer Center have found that ginger not only kills cancer cells, it also prevents them from building up resistance to cancer treatment. The American Cancer Society concurs with the University's preliminary research on animals that shows ginger may be useful in treating cancer through chemotherapy.

In a double blind, comparative test at Brigham Young University in Utah, researchers found ginger root to be more effective in coping with motion sickness than the popular over-the-counter drug Dramamine.

A Cornell University study reveals that gingerol, an active ingredient in ginger, prevents abnormal blood coagulation, guarding against heart attacks.

Ayurveda and Eating Meat

Every cell in the human body has protein. Protein helps your body to repair cells and make new ones. A balanced diet provides most healthy people with adequate protein. Protein supplements are not necessary for health.

Many people switching to an Ayurvedic lifestyle are concerned that they have to be vegetarians and will not receive the appropriate amount of protein. Ayurveda is a system of health and balance that encourages people to eat meat consciously. Conscious eating of meat means that you have honored the animal. It has had a good and nourishing life. You have expressed gratitude for its life. Buy local. Buy organic. Buy free range. Depending on your element, meat may or may not be balancing for you.

If you are The Wind, meat is balancing.
If you are The Fire, meat is not your best choice and you are best as a vegetarian.
If you are The Earth, meat should be avoided.

Meat can be balancing, but even for Wind types, it is strongly suggested that meat be consumed no more than three times per week. The problem with meat is that it is hard to digest. Ease of digestion increases your digestive fire (agni) and therefore increases metabolism. Meat is dulling to your digestive fire. It can make your stomach feel heavy and constipate you.

Red meat should be completely avoided by all doshas.

Protein Facts

In general, people need 7 grams of protein for each 20 pounds of body weight. Children, pregnant women and nursing mothers need more. That means that a 140-pound person needs 49 grams of protein.

Meat as a Source of Protein

There are pros and cons to meat as a source of protein. On the positive side, meat contains complete proteins and is therefore easier to absorb than the incomplete proteins found in nonmeat sources. A complete protein is a protein that contains the necessary amino acids to break down the protein source to facilitate absorption in the body.

However, along with absorption of protein, you are also absorbing fat when you eat meat. Meat is hard to digest and slows agni (digestive fire).

Protein Chart

SERVING SIZE (oz) PROTEIN (g)

Chick peas	7 oz.	16 g
Baked beans	8 oz.	11.5 g
Tofu	6 oz.	14 g
Milk	1/2 pint	9.2 g
Lentils	4.12 oz.	9.1 g
Soy milk	1/2 pint	8.2 g
Muesli	2.25 oz.	7.7 g
Boiled egg	1	7.5 g
Peanuts	3.5 oz.	24.3 g
Whole-grain bread	2 slices	7 g
Hard cheese	1 oz.	6.8 g
Brown rice	1 oz.	2.1 g
Broccoli	1 oz.	3.2 g
Potatoes	1 oz.	1.4 g
Soy protein pasta	1 oz.	22.75 g
Asparagus	3.5 oz.	3 g
Beans in general	3.5 oz.	9 g
Brussels sprouts	3.5 oz.	3 g
Cabbage	3.5 oz.	1 g
Carrots	3.5 oz.	.5 g
Cauliflower	3.5 oz.	3 g
Lettuce	3.5 oz.	.7 g
Mushroom	3.5 oz.	2 g
Almonds	3.5 oz.	16.9 g
Pine nuts	3.5 oz.	14 g
Sesame seeds	3.5 oz.	26.4 g
Sunflower	3.5 oz.	24 g
Spinach	3.5 oz.	2 g
Sweet corn	3.5 oz.	2.5 g
Yam	3.5	2 g
Lean meat, fish, and poultry	3.5	24.5 g

Nonmeat as a Source of Protein: Variety Is the Key

There are so many examples of nonmeat protein sources, including vegetables, legumes, seeds, nuts, fruits, whole grains, and dairy (cheese, milk, eggs, and yogurt). Whole-wheat products and vegetables are easy to digest and contain high levels of other nutrients. However, you must eat a variety of nonmeat sources to create a complete protein. This requires thought and planning. Luckily, your combining of proteins need not take place all in the same meal. You can achieve your goal throughout the day's meals.

Dairy

Is it Necessary?

For purposes the Cleanse we are eliminating dairy. Beginning right now, we will give up cow's milk for twenty-eight days. Try almond, soy, rice, or hazelnut milk instead. Slowly start to eliminate your cheese habit using the one-third withdrawal method previously described for caffeine. If you eat hard cheeses, switch to soft cheeses like feta or goat.

If you have access to non-pasteurized organic local milk (I'm talking down the street is a farmer and you walk there to pick it up daily), then you can keep your milk. Please boil the milk before you consume and add turmeric to help digest. Otherwise, try out the alternatives and see if you even notice. You may even purchase the sweetened versions.

The United States Department of Agriculture suggests daily allowances for vitamins and minerals based on the "average American." This means that some people will need that amount and some will not. Ayurveda believes each person to be unique, not average. The Wind and The Fire can consume the most dairy, as it is sweet and cooling. The Earth should not consume dairy. If you are experiencing an Earth imbalance, give up milk.

USDA Requirements for Calcium Consumption:

Age	Milligrams
4–8	800 mg
9–18	1300 mg
19–50	1000 mg
50+	1500 mg

By simply adding one glass of fortified orange juice, one glass of fortified soymilk, and one tablespoon of sesame seeds to your diet each day, you can reach 948 milligrams of calcium. Add to that some beans and leafy greens, and you are well taken care of.

Ayurveda and Milk

Dairy holds a special place in Ayurveda. Cows are considered to be sacred animals. The milk from a cow that has been well loved and well cared for rejuvenates tissues and nourishes the body. Unfortunately, these cows are few and far between in the West.

Milk is intended for those who have very strong digestion, are very sexually active, or are depleted from the force of The Wind (Vata) and need to heal, rest, and sleep. Most doshas thrive without daily dairy. If you choose to consume dairy on a regular basis, buy whole, organic, non-homogenized, and much-loved products. Homogenization changes the fat in milk and makes it very hard to digest. This encourages the accumulation of toxins, or *ama*.

Milk (post-Cleanse) should never be consumed cold. Bring it to a boil first and then turn down and let it slowly boil for five or ten minutes. This changes the molecular structure of the milk and makes it easier to digest. You may experiment with adding turmeric, cardamom, cinnamon, ginger, nutmeg, and honey to improve digestibility.

Think of milk (post-Cleanse) as a snack or a digestive aid. You can replace breakfast with warm milk adding a little bit of nutmeg, cinnamon, honey, and almonds. Warm milk taken thirty minutes before bedtime will promote sleep due to the presence of tryptophan and the heat, which raises your body's temperature. Warm milk and ghee taken prior to bedtime will aid with constipation.

Here are some more dairy facts for our Western culture:

- A high-protein diet, especially proteins from animals, causes calcium loss in the body. The proteins in cow's milk actually inhibit your body's ability to absorb calcium.
- Seventy-five percent of adults show some degree of lactase activity (lactose intolerance) worldwide.
- Jersey (small, honey-brown, friendly) cows provide the highest quality milk, but 85 percent of the milk produced in the United States is provided by Holstein cows (typical black and white cow).
- Cows are typically milked up to three times per day and given hormones, such as bsT, to boost milk production.
- Organically produced milk does use up to 80 percent more land. That's because the cows are actually getting out and enjoying life a little. If you are worried about the environment, drink less milk overall.

The following are some nondairy sources of calcium. Amounts given are in milligrams for about a one-cup serving.

Soymilk	93
Fortified soymilk	368
Quinoa	100
Mung beans	56
Baked beans	128
Navy beans	128
Refried beans	88
Bok choi	158
Turnip greens, boiled	158
Broccoli	72
French beans	111
Kelp, raw	144

Sweet potato	76
Blackberries	46
Figs	269

Processed Foods

Processed foods are any foods that have seen the inside of a factory. If you purchase food packaged in a box, can, wrapper, or bag, it is processed. When you think of processed foods, think of the following items:

- Canned food
- Frozen foods like pizza, fruit, veggies, and meats
- Foods with refined sugar (white sugar)
- Artificial sweeteners and colors
- Soft drinks and other drinks with added sugar
- Non-fresh juice
- Ready-made dinners and foods
- Instant food and soups
- Snack food like chips, crackers, and cookies

Limit your intake of processed foods during your Cleanse. We do have to continue living in the real world, so obviously we are not going to start baking our own cereals, crackers, and bread. We will not be milling our own grain and rice or drying our own beans. What this means is that you will have to choose wisely when selecting convenience foods. Shop the organic section. Look for the label "whole" on everything. Look for processed items that have the least number of ingredients. This means that they were processed the least.

Completely avoid "white" food including white sugar, white bread, white rice, white crackers, and white potatoes. White food contains a lot of refined sugar that is of no nutritional value. If you are The Earth or have an Earth imbalance in your body (you are trying to lose weight), then you need to be aware of the sugar that you are eating.

Sugar

I've spent a lot of time studying current low-carb diets to understand from an Ayurvedic perspective the connection between sugar, carbohydrates, and the fat that accumulates on your belly. I do agree that if you limit the amount of sugar and carbs in your diet, it will directly impact belly fat. I do not believe that low-carb diets are a healthy and sustainable way to live. Most low-carb diets are meat-based. While it is true that you can get all the energy you need from meat and fat, it is not a healthy plan. Meat is full of saturated fat, which is proven to cause cancer and raise LDL cholesterol. Most low-carb diets lack variety and are unsatisfying and unsustainable.

From an Ayurvedic standpoint, sugar, carbohydrates, and meat are considered sweet tastes. They are heavy and dense, and they create an overall feeling of love and satisfaction in your mind.

We crave the sweet taste as nourishment and comfort. That's why we call it comfort food. The Wind and The Fire elements can eat the sweet taste in moderation with little to no effect. The Earth element, however, cannot.

To keep it simple, incorporate the following guidelines into your life:

- If it is white, don't eat it. (Include white potatoes in this category.)
- Treat fruit as a dessert.
- Read the labels of all packaged food and check for sugar content.
- Forty grams of sugar per 2,000 calories of food is deemed safe. There is no daily recommendation for sugar.
- Avoid packaged and processed foods.

Calories

I know…I just brought up the C word. The truth is, I don't believe in counting calories. If you follow the eating routine, you will not over-consume. If you choose whole, nourishing foods of various colors with lots of spice, you will feel satisfied. It's truly that easy, and that's why I don't care about calories. However, *calorie* is a word most Americans understand, so I use it here to demonstrate how easy it is to overindulge in sugar.

The USDA provides the recommended caloric intake for sedentary and active individuals. A sedentary person does not actively exercise. An active person is a person who walks more than three miles per day at three to four miles per hour.

Sedentary/Active

Females
19–30 years of age	2,000–2,400 calories
31–50	1,800–2,200
51+	1,600–2,200

Males
19–30	2,400–3,000
31–50	2,200–3,000
51+	2,000–2,800

Remember that 40 grams of sugar per 2,000 calories is considered safe. Given this fact, this table indicates that most people should only consume 40 grams of sugar or less per day. Active men can take in closer to 60 grams. How quickly does this add up? Below is a table that I made of a day in my life (not cleansing).

4 ounce glass of organic limeade in the morning	12 grams–simple carb
1 tablespoon creamer in coffee	1 gram–simple carb
Bowl of organic cranberry ginger cereal	13 grams–complex carb

One-half cup red grapes	12 grams—simple carb
Steamed spinach	1 gram—complex carb
Scrambled egg	0 grams
Whole wheat spaghetti	1 gram—complex carb
Organic red pasta sauce	6 grams—simple carb
Broccoli	3 grams—complex carb
Glass of red wine	1 gram—simple carb
Total	50 grams

I ate pretty well that day. Still, I ended up 10 grams over what I need. That's all going straight to my belly. My big mistakes were the juice and the grapes. That's because they are high in sugar and are not a complex carb. The cereal, although high in sugar, was a good choice because it is a complex carb and I need to get 55 percent of my calories from complex carbs. Other complex carbs like whole-grain bread, pasta, and rice do not have as many sugars.

For a complete sugar table, go to www.nal.usda.gov and search for SR16. You will notice that the biggest offenders are processed foods, dried fruit, and sweet treats. Soft drinks are loaded with sugar.

Variety is the key to sustained weight control. The Cleanse will teach you how to eat a varied diet that makes sense. You will naturally begin to choose foods that have less sugar and no refined sugar.

Sugar Addiction

Sugar addiction is the most prevalent addiction in America. It is widely accepted and people tend not to take it very seriously, even though it is detrimental to a person's physical and emotional health and can lead to deeper addictions such as drugs and alcohol. Sugar is classified as addictive for the following reasons:

- It is consumed compulsively despite knowledge of its negative effects on the body.
- The neurotransmitters in your brain (dopamine and serotonin) are affected in a similar fashion to if you consume alcohol or drugs.
- Over time you build up a tolerance to sugar and must consume more to generate the same feelings.
- Over time, sugar is needed for you to feel like you are functioning normally.

Withdrawal symptoms are associated with elimination from your diet.

- Headaches
- Cravings
- Fatigue
- Tremors

- Depression
- Anxiety

If you feel that you are addicted to sugar, please read the section on dragons later in the book. As you slowly eliminate sugar from your diet, be aware of any withdrawal symptoms that you are having. Over the course of the next twenty-eight days, you will become aware of your cravings. You will become aware of your thought patterns and triggers. Your goal is to get to the root of your addiction.

May I suggest again that if you are struggling with an addiction, you should consider seeking outside counsel from a certified and trained therapist. The one-on-one counseling coupled with this program will empower you.

Alcohol

We are eliminating alcohol from our diets because it aggravates our digestive system, specifically our liver. I know that many studies indicate that consuming one drink per day in the company of others can be beneficial to your heart because it facilitates relaxation. The next twenty-eight days are about learning other techniques to relax your heart. Drinking one drink per day does not benefit your liver, even if it does benefit your heart. Alcohol puts your digestive fire out. It additionally strains your kidneys, and they are an integral part of your digestive system.

Alcohol is a depressant. One glass of wine each day can lead to depression. It may also lead to two glasses of wine each day…and then three.

Simply begin your elimination process by reducing your alcohol consumption by one third. Avoid binge drinking entirely.

What Alcohol Does to Your Digestive System

Alcohol is quickly absorbed into your bloodstream and needs very little time to digest, unlike food. Thirty percent of the alcohol you consume is expelled with breath and urine and broken down in the stomach by an enzyme called dehydrogenase. Women naturally have less of this enzyme than men, which explains why women are more quickly and adversely affected by alcohol than men. The rest of the alcohol hits the small intestine, where it is absorbed into the blood. Your liver is the next big hit, as it filters two quarts of blood per minute.

Your liver prefers to work with fatty acids, but it is smart and knows it must take care of the alcohol first, which it perceives to be poison. Yes, I said *poison.* Your liver can only digest one drink or one-half ounce of alcohol per hour. This means that your liver has to store fatty acids to break down alcohol. Many people with chronic drinking habits end up with "fatty" livers because of this. With long-term use, alcohol does irreversible damage to the cellular structure of your liver cells.

Read this twice! Once you have that drink, your liver stops digesting everything else to get the poison out. That's why that nightly glass of wine equals five to ten pounds over the course of six to eight months.

Alcohol depletes the liver, adding to weight and depressing you. Give your liver a break so that it can do its job more effectively.

Coping with a Slip

Some people slip up during the Cleanse and worry that they have ruined their Cleanse. If you slip up, it's okay. Just get back on track as soon as you realize the slip. Double your neem dosage, drink some organic orange juice, eat a banana, and make good choices, including leafy greens and fruit, for the rest of the day. Drink lots of fluid and maybe take a little aloe juice as well. This will act as a tonic and refresh your liver. Take a vitamin supplement containing all the B vitamins, and take a few doses of vitamin C.

If you know ahead of time that you will be drinking, double your neem and drink lots of water with your beverages. Always eat before imbibing to slow the absorption of the alcohol. Before you go to bed after a night on the town, boil hot water and drink a cup or two. Adding fresh ginger to your hot water is very beneficial. This will help flush your system. In the morning, take more neem, orange juice, aloe, and banana.

If you find that slipping up and drinking alcohol is a chronic problem, or if you feel that there is no way you can stop drinking for an extended period of time, then you need to ask yourself some serious questions about your alcohol consumption. Twenty-eight days is enough time to break a habit, but it is not enough time to deal with all the other aspects of what may be an addiction. We will discuss addiction further in another section. Don't stop your Cleanse. You are at a very powerful place right now.

Dealing with Cravings for Alcohol

The following steps can go a long way toward eliminating your cravings and helping you over the hump:

- Make an appointment with an acupuncturist. Tell him/her that you would like points placed in your ears that you can leave in for up to a week that help curb cravings for alcohol and sugar. (Much of our craving for alcohol stems from a craving for sugar.)
- When you are in the moment of wanting a drink, pause and ask yourself why. For me, it happens after a long day of work. I'm making dinner for the family, trying to do homework with my kids, and the phone starts ringing. A glass of wine helps me feel calmer. Unfortunately, one glass can turn into two quite easily, and that can turn into a nightly habit that ages me and adds unwanted pounds. Instead, know who you are. In this situation I need to turn off the noise, send the kids away, and take a five-minute walk or meditation. Then I can go back to my tasks, calmer and with increased focus.
- Substitute. If you are used to drinking hard alcohol, switch to wine or beer. Both are easier to digest and more filling. Dilute your wine with water, like a wine spritzer. Or even try having a glass of fruit juice in a fancy glass and pretending.
- When you are out for the evening or with friends and are being encouraged to drink, simply tell them that you are trying to lose weight. Telling people that you are trying

to lose weight deflects from their own need to drink. They will usually stop pressuring you. If they don't stop pressuring you, pretend to drink. Get a bottle of beer and carry it around all night. As long as people think you are drinking, they don't care. Remember, one in three American adults has a drinking problem, and most people don't like to drink alone. Your friends and family can sabotage you. Avoid this by following the above steps.

Additional Herbal Therapy with Alcohol

If you have been consuming one or more alcoholic beverages per day, I recommend the following additional herbal therapy:

- A multi-vitamin that includes all B-vitamins, vitamin C and D
- Flaxseed oil
- Ashwagandha
- Double your dosage of neem during your cleanse

Dragons, a Discussion on Addictions

Where you see the word *alcohol,* please feel free to substitute your personal dragon. Well-known dragons include overeating, sugar, shopping, working, gambling, sex, and drugs.

I used to start this discussion with the phrase, *There is nothing inherently wrong with consuming alcohol (substitute your dragon here).* I still believe this to be true for many people. However, recent research indicates that one in three Americans has problems stemming from alcohol abuse. One in three Americans is obese. The average household credit card debt is around $16,000, and 10 percent of adult Americans admit to being addicted to Internet pornography—28 percent of those are women. Wow! Pause here to reflect on those statistics. That's a whole lot of people suffering from abusing substances that are not "inherently" wrong.

What is substance abuse? I personally believe that substance abuse is when you consume to relieve or escape your problems, not realizing that the substance is creating those problems. That fun dragon that brings you temporary comfort starts to eat your entire life.

Perhaps you indulge your dragon because you are stressed and it relaxes you. What is stressing you? Is it your job? Is it emotions surrounding a relationship? Is it the constant demands on your life? Do you feel bad about your appearance or self? You consume and you feel better in the moment, but the next day you can't think as clearly. Your job suffers. You numb the emotions of your relationship and never have the deep meaningful conversations that need to happen or make the hard choices that you need to make. Life's demands and duties pull at you, but you buzz your time away and become inefficient at tasking. You can't stay in your moments. Your appearance continues to deteriorate as the depressive nature of most dragons pulls you down, adding wrinkles, weight, and a worn-out quality to your demeanor.

My education is grounded in spirituality. Most spiritual traditions would claim that you indulge your dragon because you are disconnected from Spirit. I do not believe this. I believe you indulge to fill the void where love is supposed to live, is hiding, or is not known. I believe you indulge to squash down fears—fear of connection, fear of betrayal, fear of the unknown, fear of failing, and fear of disappointment. These fears are founded in our childhood and in our life experiences. Once a mother, a father, a friend, a lover, or even an employer or an institution breaks your precious heart, you quickly erect barriers to entry. *Your heart is the center of existence. What wouldn't you do to protect it?*

Slay the Dragon

The following are the steps you will need to follow to slay your dragon. Do them in order. This may take a while. You may have to start over again and again until it finally sticks.

Accept

Write the following in your journal:

- Do I indulge to relieve or escape my problems?_____(yes/no)
- My problems are:
- Does my indulgence contribute to these same problems? How?
- Do I need to slay this dragon?

Commit

Write the following in your journal:

I commit to getting to know my dragon for the next twenty-eight days. I'm going to follow the plan and begin the process of getting this beast out of my life. I understand that I will have to do some soul searching and go through some emotional experiences to slay this dragon. It may be painful. I may face truths about myself that I'd rather not face. I may feel alone in this process. If I start to feel super lonely and need to talk, I'm going to reach out to someone. I may do really well for a bit of time and then slip. I'm going to forgive myself quickly if I do; it's part of the process. I've lived with this beast for way too long and I'm sick of it. I can do this.

Arm Yourself

Get someone on your side. If you are going to take the next twenty-eight days to focus on yourself and healing, then go ahead and engage a counselor to meet with you once a week for the next twenty-eight days. Often, when we start to delve deep into our psyches through the cleansing process, we need to reach out. I wish I could be there in person for you in those moments, but to be honest, I'm not a therapist. They do have a special skill set that is invaluable when you are fighting a battle with addiction.

Make an appointment with an acupuncturist and plan to have a session once a week. Acupuncture is a healing modality for addictive behavior. I have seen and heard so many success stories when the Cleanse and the services of an acupuncturist are combined.

There are also books, websites, and blogs that can support you while you slay your dragon, along with many kinds of therapies. Empower yourself with education to pick the right support structure for you.

Put Up a Defense System

Let the next twenty-eight days be all about you. This is one month that can change your life forever. Take time every day to meditate, reduce stress levels, and allow your heart to open. Journal, talk, and reach out to others. Sit with your addiction. Allow yourself to feel it in your mind and in your body. Awareness is 90 percent of your battle. Journal your cravings. Notice that your dragon does have a pattern and it is directly linked to your mind. Do your best. Do not judge yourself. If you slip, let it go and keep moving forward.

Replace your dragon with a new friend. Find a yoga studio, a spiritual center, a book club, or another activity where your mind can become stimulated and entertained again. Try something new that excites you. Reconsider the people you are hanging out with. If you are slaying alcohol, don't hang out with family and friends that overindulge. If you are slaying sugar, avoid the friends that share your addiction. Become a guardian of your journey and embrace all that you are going through.

Routines for Eating and Living

Eating and Daily Routine...Goals to Reach For

- Eat three meals a day around the same times each day. This is a critical success factor. The idea is to train your body when to digest and to take advantage of the natural rhythms of the day when digestion is highest.
- Include the colors of the rainbow in your meals. This will ensure that you are finding satisfaction in your meals and receiving all the nutrition that you require. Do think of adding spices to your meals to color them. Spicy spices promote digestion and detoxification.
- Breakfast should be eaten within one hour of rising and preferably before 8:00 a.m. If you normally skip breakfast, try the Yogi Breakfast recipe. It's fast, easy, and delicious. You can make it in less than five minutes and drink it in your car on your way to work. Better still is to sit down and simply enjoy it.
- Lunch should be your largest meal. If you are eating meat, consume it at lunch instead of breakfast or dinner. Your digestion is strongest at lunch. The natural rhythm of the planet and of you is to be heated up the most when the sun is highest in the sky.
- Set the atmosphere:
  Sit down to eat. Sometimes this means pulling off the road and eating quietly in your car.
  Set a pleasant table, even when dining alone.
  Eat in silence or listen to nice calming music.
  Eat in the company of others discussing light happy topics. Never argue or discuss deep emotional issues during a meal.

- If you must drink with your meal, then sip room temperature water. Think of your digestion as a fire. You don't want to put anything in your stomach that puts out your fire. Iced beverages douse your fire. It is best not to drink with your meals. Let your food take up three-fourths of your stomach and leave room for your digestive juices. If you must drink, drink after you eat.

- A meal, for the purposes of cleansing, is the size of your two fists put together. Literally make two fists and hold them up to your food. If you have more than the size of your two fisted hands, you have too much. (For clarity, I'm not talking about the inside of your fist. I'm talking about the size of your fisted hand, which is about 1 cup per hand, for a total of a little less than 2 cups). Leave one-fourth of your stomach empty to digest.

- Eat slowly and chew your food thoroughly. This starts the digestive process. Consider counting your chews. Twenty-five times is best for optimal digestion. Put your fork down between bites and focus on the flavors and sensations of each bite.

- Never talk with your mouth full, and please chew your food with your mouth closed. This will help to reduce gas and bloating, not to mention it's just polite.

- If you are eating out, share a meal. Favor vegetables and whole grains. Avoid white pastas and creamy sauces. The spicier, the better. Think Japanese, Thai, Indian, Mexican, or Italian. Avoid "American" restaurants.

- Go for a ten-minute walk after you eat. Seriously, that's walking five minutes one way and turning around and walking five minutes back. You can do it.

- Avoid snacking during your cleanse. If you find that you must snack, you'll find a few "snack-like" items in this book to tide you over as you slowly eliminate this habit.

Daily Routine...Nature's Rhythms

- Before you go to bed each night, place a glass of water on your bedside table.
- Get up each morning between 5:00 and 7:00 a.m.
- Before you get out of bed, drink that glass of water down.
- Go to the bathroom and sit on the toilet with the intention to eliminate. You may or may not go, but set the intention. Eventually, you will be able to get up first thing in the morning and eliminate all of the digested food before your body starts to reabsorb the waste.
- Brush your teeth, then let your dogs out or do what you have to do with the noisemakers in your house to quiet them.
- Do a little yoga or walking. Even just five minutes will get you circulating and your mind clear.
- Meditate. Note that this is an Earth period and your thoughts are calm. It's the best time to meditate.
- Perform your oil massage before or after your shower.

- Go about your day, taking advantage of any opportunity to spend time in nature and to be in silence. Drive with the radio off, turn your cell phone off, avoid the TV, and avoid crowded spaces.
- Meditate as the sun goes down. (Notice that you are in an Earth phase again after 6:00 p.m. and your thoughts are naturally calm.)
- Take your herbs before bedtime.
- Bedtime is around 10:00 p.m. No TV is allowed in bed. Read something spiritual.

The Times of Day When the Doshas Are Most Active

This information can guide you to appropriately use the energies of the doshas to support you in activity.

6:00 a.m.–10:00 a.m.: The Earth (Kapha)

This is a hypometabolic period and the best time to perform exercises. This is especially true if you want to lose weight. If you are trying to heal your body, this is a good time to take medicine. This is also a great time to meditate.

10:00 a.m.–2:00 p.m.: The Fire (Pitta)

This is the time when you are transforming. Your agni (digestive fire) is highest at this time. This is the best time for you to eat a large meal, meaning lunch.

2:00 p.m.–6:00 p.m.: The Wind (Vata)

This is a hypermetabolic period. This is when you want to do all of your thinking and work that requires thought and creativity. Your mind is moving fast.

6:00 p.m.–10:00 p.m.: The Earth (Kapha)

This is when we slowly wind down from the day. By ten o'clock, you are ready for bed. Wind down with some reading and entertainment. This is a great time to meditate.

10:00 p.m.–2:00 a.m.: The Fire (Pitta)

You are asleep and your body is digesting and healing. Your body is rejuvenating itself and detoxifying. This is a very important time to be asleep and healing—renew and detox and sleep.

2:00 a.m.–6:00 a.m.: The Wind (Vata)

You slowly become hypermetabolic. This is when you have periods of REM sleep. You may find that this is the period of time when your sleep becomes interrupted. Clear mental stress.

Get up at 6:00 a.m. and no later than 7:00 a.m.

This is when you will feel the freshest and most alert. Drink your warm water to start the process of digestion. This is a signal to your body. Brush your teeth, and scrape your tongue.

Self-Administered Oil Massage, or Abhyanga

Translated *abhyanga* means "loving hands." Abhyanga may be the best thing that has come from Ayurveda. It combines oils that are nutritive to your body with touch that soothes your mind and spirit. It is easy, inexpensive, and healing. Once you begin an abhyanga practice, you will make it part of your daily routine with effortless ease.

An oil massage is the perfect way to start and end your day. It is a self-massage that can be performed to invigorate you in the morning and relax you in the evening. It only takes two to ten minutes to perform and provides immeasurable healing benefits.

Oil is better for your skin than lotion. Unlike lotion, oil is fat-soluble and is absorbed by your cells. The tiny capillaries on your skin absorb the oil into your bloodstream and distribute it throughout your nervous and lymphatic systems. Additionally, oils can have a calming or an invigorating effect when treated with different herbs. For example, lavender-infused oil relaxes you. Cinnamon-infused oil invigorates you.

Your body is in constant dynamic exchange with the environment. You are quite literally digesting your environment. It is recommended to use products that you can actually eat.

Oils by Body Type Post Cleanse

These oils are all wonderful carrier oils that can be used daily. If you wish, you may infuse them with other essential oils. Please note that sesame seed oil is the perfect oil for the Cleanse. It is warming and grounding to The Wind (Vata) on your skin. If you want to get creative or do not like the smell of sesame oil, consider the alternatives offered below by body and mind type.

Base Oils by Element
The Wind

Sesame
Avocado
Peanut
Walnut
Castor
Flax

Note: The Wind (Vata) causes dryness in skin. Sesame oil post-cleanse is the best!

The Fire

Coconut
Sunflower
Olive
Grapeseed

Note: The Fire (Pitta) causes dull oily skin. Coconut oil post-cleanse is the best!

The Earth

Almond
Safflower
Mustard
Corn

Canola
Soy

Note: The Earth (Kapha) causes thickness and puffiness. Almond oil post-cleanse is the best!

All
Jojoba
Primrose
Hazelnut
Aloe
Wheat germ

Essential Oils by Element (Twelve Drops of Essential Oil per One Ounce of Carrier Oil)

The Wind (warming & nourishing)

Bergamot
Orange
Sandalwood
Frankincense
Camphor
Turmeric
Neroli
Ylang Ylang
Cinnamon
Musk
Vanilla
Lavender

The Fire (cooling & soothing)

Lily
Honeysuckle
Sandalwood
Mint
Lemongrass
Gardenia
Neroli
Jasmine
Lavender
Chamomile

The Earth (warming & stimulating)

Bergamot

Orange
Peppermint
Frankincense
Camphor
Turmeric
Pine
Jasmine
Lavender
Chamomile
Eucalyptus
Sage

All (tri-dosha)
Tea Tree
Rose

The Massage

The oil massage should be performed on a towel, as it can be messy. You may warm the oil by simply running under hot water or taking it into the shower with you. (This conserves water too). You may consider purchasing an oil warmer. Simply put the oil on to heat before you get in your shower and it will be ready when you come out. The massage should take five to ten minutes.

Most people prefer to perform the massage prior to showering to avoid feeling oily throughout the day. At bedtime, however, plan to leave the oil on to absorb and heal while you sleep.

Start at your scalp. Use a couple of tablespoons of oil and vigorously massage your scalp in small circles. Work your way down to your ears and massage the inside and outside of your ears.

Move to your face. Massage in little gentle circles going clockwise. The carrier oils are perfect for your face. Most oils, in fact, are antibacterial and anti-inflammatory and can therefore benefit skin that is prone to eruptions. I use sesame oil to take off my makeup.

Move to your arms and legs. Vigorously rub the oil in long strokes. Some say that if you rub upwards, it will break down cellulite…no proof on that yet though!

Rub your torso in a clockwise circular motion. (You are the clock.) Enlist a friend to do the hard to reach places! Remember, this is healing touch therapy.

The Touch Research Institute in conjunction with Duke University found that after massage, the human body secretes lower levels of the stress hormones cortisol, norepinephrine, and dopamine.

A 1996 study published in the *International Journal of Neuroscience* found that massaged subjects completed math problems in significantly less time—and with a whole lot fewer errors—than test subjects who were not massaged.

According to the ancient science of Ayurveda, oil rubbed into the skin provides numerous benefits:

1. Prevents dehydration; strengthens the nerves
2. Creates an electrochemical balance in the body
3. Soothes insomnia
4. Nourishes the body, promotes steadiness and confidence
5. Promotes good vision
6. Heals and prevents nervous system imbalances
7. Alleviates fatigue and stress from overworking
8. Increases longevity and reverses aging
9. Strengthens the electromagnetic field of the body
10. Creates a protective shield around the body against negativity
11. Increases the immune system
12. Stimulates antibody production

Why I Love Sesame Oil

Sesame is considered *sattvic* in Ayurvedic terms, meaning it is pure. Sesame seed oils have been used for thousands of years in the Vedic tradition. The nutritional impact of sesame seeds is impressive. I highly recommend adding one ounce of sesame seeds to your daily diet. The following table shows the nutritional content in one-fourth cup of sesame seeds.

Nutrient	Amount	Percent of Daily Value
Copper	1.48 mg	74%
Manganese	0.88 mg	44%
Tryptophan	120 mg	37.5%
Calcium	351 mg	35.1%
Magnesium	126 mg	31.6%
Iron	5.24 mg	29.1%
Phosphorus	226 mg	22%
Zinc	2.8 mg	18.7%
Vitamin B1 (Thiamin)	0.28 mg	18.7%
Dietary fiber	4.24 g	17%
Calories	206	

For thousands of years, sesame oil has been used in holistic healing. It naturally possesses the properties of an antibacterial, an antifungal, an antiviral and an anti-inflammatory. Experiments with sesame oil are now focused on its antibacterial properties in fighting staphylococcus and streptococcus. It is also used in the treatment of athlete's foot, hepatitis, diabetes, and migraines. Used in vitro, it has inhibited the growth of malignant melanoma and inhibited the replication of colon cancer cells.

Sesame oil is a potent antioxidant that neutralizes oxygen radicals in the tissues beneath the skin. Sesame oil enters the bloodstream quickly through the capillaries on the surface of the skin. It aids in maintaining good cholesterol (HDL) and lowering bad cholesterol (LDL).

Because the oil is a cell growth regulator, it slows down the degeneration of cells. It provides valuable fat to the cells it is nourishing in the small and large intestines.

Sesame oil has been used as a mouth rinse and reduces the bacteria that cause gingivitis by 85 percent. It has been used as nose drops to treat chronic sinusitis. Used as a throat gargle, it destroys strep and other common cold bacteria.

If you are suffering from psoriasis or dry skin, it acts as an emollient to sooth and lubricate.

It is a natural UV (SPF of 4) protector and, if used after exposure to the sun and wind, it will alleviate the symptoms of sunburn. Additionally, it can protect the skin from the harmful effects of chlorine in a pool.

Sesame oil is highly recommended for the following conditions:

- Chronic cough
- Weak lungs
- Chronic constipation
- Hemorrhoids
- Dysentery
- Amenorrhea
- Dysmenorrheal
- Receding gums
- Tooth decay
- Hair loss
- Weak bones
- Osteoporosis
- Emaciation
- Convalescence

How does sesame oil act, and what does it do?

- Rejuvenate
- Demulcent
- Emollient
- Nutritive tonic
- Laxative
- Antibacterial

- Antifungal
- Antiviral

Sleeping

Routine for all

- Arise between 5:00 and 7:00 a.m. all seven days of the week.
- Bedtime is between 10:00 and 11:00 p.m. Read a nice, uplifting book until sleepy.
- Do not watch TV in your bedroom.
- Keep your bedroom very cool, with lots of comfy covers.
- Before you go to bed each night, place a glass of water on your bedside table. In the morning, drink the water.
- If you are female, lie on your left side to sleep. If you are male, lie on your right side. Before falling asleep:

  Recapitulate your day. Start at the beginning of the day and quickly walk through the day's events. Just observe them. This should only take a few minutes. If you get "stuck" on an event, simply allow the emotions to arise and observe the emotion. Do this in a clinical and analytical fashion. Before you go to sleep, tell yourself that you will remember your dreams. As you prepare to fall asleep, imagine a pure white light in your heart center. This is your divine essence. Allow it to grow and flood your body and your room. Just imagine it…imagine it heals you. If you wake in the middle of the night, do this again. Keep a journal by your bed to write down any dreams or insights you have had during the night.

The National Foundation for Sleep's definition of sufficient sleep is "a sleep duration that is followed by a spontaneous awakening and leaves one feeling refreshed and alert for the day." This agrees with the Ayurvedic definition of adequate sleep, and the statement is profound in that it allows for the fact that different elements will need different amounts of sleep.

Side effects of insufficient sleep include the following:

- Increased heart rate
- Increased blood pressure
- Increased inflammation leading to coronary artery disease
- Impaired glucose tolerance (diabetes)
- Increased hunger/appetite (obesity)
- Increased risk of hypertension
- Weight gain

When to Sleep

Nighttime is the best time to sleep. Around 6:00 p.m., we naturally start to wind down as the energy of The Earth (Kapha) settles over our region of the world. Our mind settles during this time. This period lasts from 6:00 p.m. to 10:00 p.m. Intend to be in bed by 10:00 p.m.

Beginning around 10:00 p.m., the energy of The Fire (Pitta) comes into play. This period lasts from 10:00 p.m. to 2:00 a.m. During this period, your body is very active, healing itself and digesting food. If you regularly stay up later than 10:00 p.m., you are interrupting this critical time to heal and digest. Also, this period *is* an active period. That means that if you are not settled in bed, your mind, which was settled by the energy of The Earth, may become very active again, interfering with your ability to go to sleep.

Around 2:00 a.m., the energy of The Wind (Vata) moves in. This is the perfect time for your emotional body to heal as you enter a serene and luminous sleep. Your dreams become vivid and your mind is allowed to play out not just its fantasies, but its worries and anxieties as well. You problem solve while you sleep.

The Earth (Kapha):	6:00 p.m.–10:00 p.m.:	your mind settles
The Fire (Pitta):	10:00 p.m.–2:00 a.m.:	your body digests
The Wind (Vata):	2:00 a.m.–6:00 a.m.:	your emotions process

If You Are The Wind

You must begin your bedtime routine by 10:00 p.m. Staying up late greatly aggravates you, and you will miss out on that good energy of The Earth that slows your mind. Arise by 7:00 a.m. each morning.

If You Are The Fire

You must begin your bedtime routine between 10:00 p.m. and 11:00 p.m. Staying up late greatly aggravates you because by midnight, it is full Fire time. You may find that you get the munchies or even experience a sour belly as the gastric juices in your system heat up. Do not eat two hours prior to bedtime.

If You Are The Earth

You may go to bed between 10:00 p.m. and 11:30 p.m. The Earth generally does not have any problems falling asleep, and your bedtime routine may not need to include the relaxation of meditation, yoga nidra, or reading something pure (sattvic). In fact, The Earth likes to sleep in excess. You are the element that needs to force yourself out of bed in the morning. Getting up between 5:00 a.m. and 6:00 a.m. each day is beneficial, especially if you are trying to lose weight.

Bedtime Routine

It is beneficial to have a nightly routine for bed. It stimulates a relaxation response in your mind. Here is a simple plan:

- Brush your teeth with Neem toothpaste and floss.
- Scrape your tongue with a tongue scraper.

- Wash face, hands, and feet.
- Massage your face, hands, and feet with sesame oil.
- Meditate for ten to fifteen minutes in your meditation spot (not in bed).
- Turn your lights low and light a relaxing scent such as lavender, sandalwood, or ylang ylang.
- Yoga nidra is beneficial. You may want to purchase a guided CD to assist you.
- If you are going to read, read something spiritual or inspirational.

Sleep Aids

Routine, meditation, and yoga nidra are your best sleep aids. Herbal supplements like Valerian and Kava Kava are also beneficial at night. The herb Ashwaganda promotes restful sleep but does not make you sleepy. It simply calms and nourishes you throughout your day, and you will find that you sleep more easily as your thought process is settled.

If you are Cleansing from using other pharmaceutical sleep aids, consider adding Valerian to your weaning process. Learn more at **www.elementalom.com**.

Warm milk does facilitate sleep. The warmth of the milk raises your body's temperature, promoting relaxation. Milk contains tryptophan, which is also found in those Thanksgiving turkeys that make us so sleepy.

Aromatherapy to Promote Relaxation and Sleep

Place a few drops of any of these essential oils on your pillow, burn incense, or infuse your sesame oil with these scents.

- Chamomile
- Clary sage
- Geranium
- Lavender
- Mandarin
- Marjoram
- Neroli
- Rose
- Sandalwood

Napping

The general rule is no napping, especially during the Cleanse. Napping increases the force of The Earth (Kapha) in your body and creates dullness and lethargy. The Earth (Kapha) especially should not nap…I know you want to all the time, but it is very bad for you. You have a lot of very grounded energy in your mind and body already. Napping increases this energy and makes you dull and lethargic. There are a few exceptions to this rule, however. The Wind (Vata) may take catnaps, but they should not exceed ten minutes. Also, during Fire (Pitta) season, when it is hot outside, all elements may nap for extended periods of time, as the intensity of the heat tends to drain all energy.

Napping is recommended for any of the following situations, but naps should not exceed fifteen minutes and should be taken in the afternoon.

- Children
- Elderly
- Exhaustion
- Overindulgence in intoxicants, work, sex, or physical exertion
- Trauma or grief
- Travel or excessive running of errands and chores

Sleeping Positions

Believe it or not, from a yogic perspective, sitting up is the best way to sleep. Many yogis will alternate sleeping and meditating all night long. I don't recommend you try this during the Cleanse. Once you are firmly grounded in your meditation and yogic practices, you will decide this on your own. For now, lie down to sleep.

The question of why we roll to our right side when we end Shavasana often comes up. Shavasana is the corpse pose performed at the end of every yoga class. Your yoga teacher will rouse you quietly from your Shavasana and ask you to roll to your right in a fetal position. When you are on your right side, you will find it to be most relaxing. This opens your left nostril, or the Nadi Ida. It activates the right hemisphere of your brain. This side of your brain is more feminine, more emotional, and more peaceful, and it resonates with the lunar energy of the moon. This is the part of your brain that understands you are part of a bigger whole. You are a soul in a soup of the One Soul. This side does not understand your "I am-ness." It doesn't understand ego. The right side of your body is the best side to sleep on, especially if you have trouble sleeping.

Lying on your left side opens your right nostril, the Nadi Pingala. It activates the left hemisphere of your brain. This side of your brain is more masculine and more active, and it resonates with the solar energy of the sun. Language lives in the left side. The left hemisphere analyzes the situation, determines the risk, and formulates logical strategy. This is the part of your brain that is ego-obsessed. It identifies with itself and keeps you separate from the others. The left side is the best side to sleep on if you find that you are not enjoying pleasures of the senses such as food and sex or if you are feeling shy and passive.

Lying on your back or stomach is not a good way to sleep. On your back, your energy dissipates and leaves. Lying on your stomach, you cannot breath effectively.

Meditation: The Most Important Practice of The Cleanse

The practice of sitting quietly in what is commonly known as meditation is the foundation for success in this program. During meditation we learn to quiet our minds, observe our thoughts, replace our thoughts, and control our minds.

Depending on your dosha, it is estimated that you have between sixty and ninety thousand thoughts a day. The vast majority of these thoughts consist of dwelling on the past or worrying about the future. The past is gone. It's done. The future is uncertain. You just can't know. That means you are doing a lot of thinking that is causing you stress. Do you realize that 90 percent of disease is caused by stress? It isn't caused by soft drinks, fast food, or spending hours in front of the TV. Stress is caused by negative thinking patterns. Of course, I would argue that because you are stressed, you are making some of those poor nutritional and lifestyle choices.

Meditation has been studied in the United States since the Beatles popularized transcendental meditation in the '60s. If you want to get to the clinical realities of meditation, please search Harvard Medical School, the Cleveland Clinic, and the Mayo Clinic in conjunction with the term *meditation* on your browser. The facts are in: people who meditate are smarter, appear younger, and seem happier than those who do not. Why?

The reasons are simple. In meditation, you learn to control your thoughts. As you sit in meditation, you will become distracted by your thoughts. Your thoughts will begin to annoy you as you realize that you are obsessed over something that happened long ago, you worry about your future, or you speak poorly to yourself. You might find that you are very negative, critical, or judgmental.

As your annoyance grows, you will desire to break free from these negative thought patterns and replace them with silence, joy, and positive thinking. Through meditation, your awareness of your thinking will be brought into your day-to-day activities. You will find yourself stopping your negative thoughts and replacing those thoughts with awareness. You will learn to respond instead of react.

In the silence of meditation practice, you become so quiet that you eventually experience a tangible spiritual connection. This is a state of bliss that is a reward of regular meditation practice. It is a gift given to the quiet mind. You will feel a divine peace and connection to everything and everyone around you. It is a very pleasant and powerful feeling. Through this connection, you will discover your heart's desires and connect with your life's purpose. It is often said that when you pray, you are talking to God. When you meditate, you are listening.

The Practice

Make a promise to yourself to spend time each morning practicing your meditation. We choose to practice meditation in the morning because it is an Earthy time of day. The Earth grounds our thoughts, and we are more receptive to the practice. This may mean that you get up earlier before your family stirs. Be comfortable. Be alone. Be in silence.

There are many ways to meditate. Anything that you have one pointed focus on can become a meditation. This includes eating, walking, washing the dishes, and practicing yoga. Yoga defined is one pointed attention on anything of your choosing. Some people choose to stare at the flame of a candle or at a beautiful picture. Some people listen to music.

I don't want you to practice any of these methods unless it is simply for fun. For the Cleanse, you will be practicing mantra meditation. The word *mantra* translates from the Sanskrit to "instrument of the mind." A mantra is simply a word or phrase that you say over and over again to give your mind something to do other than think thoughts.

I think of a mantra as a little toy that I give my brain to distract my mind from having other thoughts. You will notice that your mind is very much like a little puppy. It wants to go play, so you must entertain it. The most common and widely used mantra is "so hum." It translates from the Sanskrit as "I am." If you do not feel comfortable using Sanskrit, feel free to use the English. I find, however, that the mantra connects nicely and effortlessly with the breath.

Getting Started

- Begin your morning with ten to fifty minutes of yoga. Sun salutations are perfect. You can go to www.elementalom.com to view the practice. Connect your movement to breath. Take a small Shavasana, or relaxation.
- Sitting comfortably and quietly, close your eyes.
- Breathe in and out through your nose.
- Take seven deep breaths in and deep breaths out to relax. This is the only manipulation of your breath. After seven breaths, let it go back to its natural rhythm.
- Roll your head around if you need to. Get all your fidgeting out.
- Notice your breath. Do not manipulate your breath. Simply notice that it comes in through your nose and out through your nose. Your breath is natural. There is no manipulation of the breath. It simply comes in and goes out.
- Notice the noises and smells in your environment. Accept that they are part of the meditation.
- As you breathe in, think the word *so* or *I*.
- As you breath out, think the word *hum* or *am*.
- Stay with your mantra and just let your breath flow naturally.
- As you notice thoughts, simply acknowledge them and pull your mind back to your mantra. Accept that the thoughts that arise are part of your meditation.
- Treat your brain kindly, just like you would a puppy. If it wants to roam, give it its toy (the mantra).

Three Things That May Happen During Your Practice

1. You may fall asleep. If you fall asleep, that is okay. It just means you are tired. Reconsider your routine and how you might adjust it to accommodate your body's need to rest. Make sure you are not lying down to meditate. It is possible to fall asleep sitting up, but that won't happen very often, as it is quite startling.
2. You may think thoughts. If you think thoughts, that is okay, too. Perhaps you have a lot on your mind and need to think thoughts. The practice of meditation includes thinking

thoughts. Consider for a moment that your mantra is simply another thought. It is a directed and controlled thought of your choosing. Each time you realize you are thinking thoughts, gently bring yourself back to your mantra. Remember that this is a meditation *practice*. Meditation is a reward that comes from practice. You may consider journaling prior to meditating to get thoughts out.

3.   You may experience thoughtlessness. You may emerge from your meditation surprised at how quickly time has passed. That just means you were meditating. Congrats!

When you are done meditating, give yourself a few minutes to slowly open your eyes and bring yourself back to consciousness. Relax for five or ten minutes prior to beginning your day. Lying down and covering up is always encouraged. Journaling your experience is also encouraged.

Meditating is powerful—you will begin to process emotional situations from your past. This is good. You may question your life and its purpose. This is also good. You may experience great extremes of emotion. Just acknowledge that you are healing and let the emotions pass. Do not judge yourself.

Frequently Asked Questions About Meditation

Why won't my thoughts settle down?

They will eventually, but they will never permanently settle. Remember, your thoughts are part of the meditation practice. Simply observe them and go back to your mantra over and over. It will take at least twenty-one days to establish your practice. Be patient.

Meditating first thing in the morning before your day begins keeps the "I have to do this and that" thinking at bay. Doing sun salutations with breath awareness will get your body and mind in a settled state to receive meditation. I can't stress enough how effective it is to move your body prior to meditation. Yoga is perfect, but going for a quick walk will clear your mind as well.

It is effective to journal prior to meditating. Simply go to your journal and write one to three pages of anything that comes up. Literally dump all of your thoughts out into your journal. I call these "Fire pages." They do not have to make sense. They do not have to be linked or logical. Spelling does not matter. This is not a story or a journal entry you will ever read again. This is a brain dump to get the frenzy out.

Purchase the book *Yoga Nidra* by Dr. Richard Miller. In the back of the book is a CD. Simply lie on the floor in a comfy position and listen to the guided meditation. This will get you in touch with your physical, subtle, and spiritual bodies. You will find that it is very engaging and will give you desire to connect. Do this every day and then come to a seated position to do your meditation. Your mind will quiet. Another side effect is you will sleep better.

Honor that sometimes you need to think. Even if you have been practicing for a very long time and have an established meditation practice, things in life will come up and your mind will want to play in the details. For me, I find that I have many creative ideas and projects that throw my meditation off because I get so excited about them. When it becomes overwhelming and none of the above works, I just allow myself to think. Eventually I get bored with it and my mind settles. I call this "sitting with my thoughts." It is a practice in mindfulness, and I do not teach it as a meditation technique. It is a beautiful way to honor your monkey mind in thought-filled moments and to avoid frustration.

If you are having trouble quieting your thoughts, please consider if you are following your spiritual routine. Ask yourself if you are spending adequate time in silence. Quiet your life down and say no to activities and events. If you do these things you will have much less clutter to think about.

Why am I am so emotional when I meditate? I find myself crying.

Raw emotions and crying are very common. When I first began my meditation practice I was meditating twice a day for forty minutes each session. For the first three months of this practice, I simply cried and brought myself back to my mantra over and over. I did not experience a meditative state for those first three months. That's 120 hours of crying.

I needed to cry. I was in chronic pain from a back injury. My life and my marriage were falling apart. I was losing it. Those first three months of my practice allowed me time to pay attention to my emotional and physical pain. It allowed me time to figure out what I wanted in life. It allowed me time to find myself again. After 120 hours of crying, I started to make good choices and to get happy, and I experienced a meditative state. It was worth all the crying.

Meditation is a safe place to honor your feelings as they come up. So often, we shove emotions like anger, betrayal, fear, and disappointment deeply down inside of us. When we get really quiet, they bubble up. Just sit with the emotions and allow yourself to finally feel them and begin to process them. Know that emotions have a path to follow. Deep down, we are all starting with fear. Fear moves to pain, pain moves to anger, anger moves to sadness, sadness becomes compassion, and that ultimately becomes forgiveness. If you are sitting in anger, be angry and know that you will move to sad and so on. We must honor our emotions. Shoving them down and hoping they go away doesn't work.

Many of you have probably been reading spiritual books that encourage you to simply observe your emotions. This is not a yogic process. Yoga honors the emotions and expresses the emotions. You are here to live. Living is feeling. If you feel anger, it's important to be angry. Talk, write, and think about it until your anger turns to sadness. Get it out. Of course, you want to get it out in a sattvic (pure) way. Don't explode all over everyone. Find a constructive way to express.

I've been meditating for a long time, and I have an understanding of my emotions. That doesn't mean that emotions don't come up. I've simply learned to choose to respond to them in a positive way. When I feel jealous, I sit with it and ask myself why. When I become angry, I sit with it and work through the problem to a positive solution.

Enhance the meditation process with journaling and reading inspirational books and literature. Immerse yourself in the process of understanding your emotions and finding compassion around the situations that come up. I want to remind you how beneficial it can be to seek spiritual or psychological counseling as part of your initial journey into meditation. This program, in conjunction with counseling, can allow you to conquer the negative emotions that have been pulling you down your whole life.

Why do I fall asleep?

You must be tired. Look at how you are living. Are you following nature's routine? Do you get in bed by 10:00 p.m. and get up by 6:00 or 7:00 a.m.? Allow yourself a ten-minute rest after your meditation to reward yourself.

Make sure you aren't meditating lying down or in bed. Is your chair too comfortable? Are you very warm and cozy? Make sure you are seated comfortably at a nice temperature, but not so warm it lulls you to sleep. Practice yoga for 10 minutes before you meditate. This will enliven you with breath and get your muscles happy.

Why can't I find the time to meditate?

Remember that we scheduled time into your day when you began the Cleanse. What is going on in your life that you can't spend some quality time on yourself? What needs to go? Meditation is a critical success factor to your Cleanse.

Meditation creates time. In fact, many yogis develop magical powers called *siddhis* as their meditation progresses. Although creation of time is not classically defined as a siddhi, I like to think of it as a magical yogi superpower. When you sit down to meditate, everything becomes clear. If my mind is jumping from thing to thing and I cannot focus because I have so much to do and my brain is on overload, that's when I stop and go sit in my chair. In my chair, my mind settles, things organically prioritize, and magically my to do list rearranges. I leave my chair focused, centered, and streamlined. I become an efficient thinking machine and I stop wasting time. You are wasting time not meditating.

Are you avoiding your meditation because it makes you mentally or emotionally uncomfortable? Perhaps you are uneasy because of your emotional response to meditation. This could be the first time in years that you have allowed yourself to slow and sit with your emotions. It can be a little scary. Know that at the end of twenty-eight days you are going to have shifted through many of your emotions and habits. Make meditation, journaling, and processing your emotions a priority.

Why is my body so uncomfortable when I meditate?

If your body is uncomfortable due to illness, injury, disease, stress, or weight, then you will have a hard time meditating until you can get your discomfort under control. Do not give up. Oddly, meditation is the cure for what is making you too uncomfortable to meditate.

For this reason, Cleansers meditate in conjunction with daily walking, yoga, nutritional guidance, and emotional exercises to relieve stress. It is a process that in combination will facilitate your comfort in meditation.

Stick with your meditation practice. Make yourself as comfortable as possible. When your mind wanders to an ache or pain, simply sit with it. Notice it. Send your breath to fill up the space, and imagine releasing the discomfort with your out breath. Gently pull your mind back to your mantra. Throughout your day, send breath to your discomfort. Start to pay attention to when you feel the most discomfort. Is it stress-related? Is it at a certain time of the day?

Begin to treat your discomfort as a visiting guest. It's there. It needs attention, and it will be leaving soon.

Why are my friends, family, and/or coworkers discouraging me from doing this practice?

You are starting to do something healthy and positive for yourself. You are probably excited. You may already be feeling the amazing healing benefits, and you want to share them with everyone. That's natural, but I strongly encourage you to stop talking about your experience. Your friends and family may mistake your excitement as a message that you want them to change what *they* are doing and join you. Simply enjoy the experience and your better health. Your friends, family, and coworkers will eventually notice that you are glowing and happy, and they will ask you what you are doing. Then you can tell them.

I'm worried that meditation interferes with my religion. Does it?

Never do anything that doesn't resonate with you. We live in an age in which we are learning to listen to ourselves. If you feel in your heart that meditation is not right for you, then it isn't. Before you make your decision, however, seek counsel with your religious leader and with yourself.

As an advocate for meditation and for connection to Spirit in any form, I would strongly urge you to think of meditation and religion separately. I think of a religious center as a great place to connect with others and to hear a positive message. It is a sanctuary for prayer and communion. I have a practice of praying to God, and I do believe there is great power in group prayer.

Meditation, on the other hand, is very personal and private. In meditation, I connect with myself and with Spirit. It's a more one-on-one relationship with what I perceive to be God. Each person's idea of *Spirit* may be different depending on religious beliefs and upbringing. There are seven billion people on the planet and seven billion ways to heaven. In meditation, there is room for all beliefs. If you want to look at it purely through a clinical view, you are sitting with your own personal thoughts and learning to control your thoughts. You are learning to stay in your present moments and enjoy them. You are learning to think with a positive and happy view. Religion does not need to be involved in any of that.

I do not believe in Spirit or God. Will meditation work for me?

Do you believe that you are sitting here right now reading this? (I'm going to assume you said yes). That's all you need. If you don't want to connect to Spirit, then think of meditation as a time to simply connect to yourself. After all, you know that you are real.

Make Time to Meditate

Write down your current schedule of activities between 6:00 a.m. to 11:00 p.m., Monday through Sunday. Find one to three things that you do every day at the same time, for example, (1) getting up, (2) eating a meal, and (3) going to bed. Plan to pair your meditation with one of these activities that are already routine for you.

Creating a Sacred Space in Your Home

Everything you feel, see, and touch is an extension of your spirit. Surrounded by beauty and tranquility, your spirit flourishes. Make your home feel like a sanctuary by creating a sacred space to nourish your body, calm your mind, and awaken your spirit.

Do what you can now to create your sanctuary. When I first began meditating, I sat on the couch in the living room. This worked well because I would get up very early, before my family, and only the cat would interrupt. The couch happened to have bolster pillows to offer good lower back support and my living room had very little clutter and a natural Zen quality.

I found, however, that as I embraced my spiritual lifestyle more and more I began to accumulate books to study, artifacts from retreats and workshops, incense, shawls, and blankets. I also noticed that if I had a yoga rug handy I could do a few sun salutations and then slip into meditation more comfortably. My grandmother passed away and left me a knitted blanket of hot pink and green that I loved to cover myself in during my meditation, even though it clashed entirely with my living room. I didn't want to travel from one room to the next or pack up my books to keep the living room as it was.

I moved to a closet. Seriously. My house at the time had a large storage space with a window off of the guest room. I cleaned all of the junk out, bought a beautiful meditation chair, and filled up the space with my knitted blanket and artifacts. In one corner were a yoga mat, blocks, and other props. In another was a twin mattress with a groovy bedspread where I could nap and read. The room also held an altar, my spiritual books, and some mementos. Over time, I added a reiki timer, a CD player, and mandalas for the walls. It probably looked like a college dorm room from the '60s, but I loved everything about it.

I live in a different home now, and I have an entire room dedicated to my spiritual practice. The furniture has been upgraded from the dormitory look. I still have the same beautiful meditation chair, but it now sits on a fur rug created by a Native American artisan. My room is full of artwork and gifts given to me and smells of jasmine. My altar is much larger to accommodate my growing collection of statues and candles. The room seems to grow and change with me. Sometimes books are piled about, sometimes I clean everything out of the room so only my chair rests in there.

I love that room so much. When I walk into it, I immediately begin to settle. The scent alone, which is sacred to only that room of my house, starts my relaxation. My family knows that this is a special room. I invite my children to join me occasionally and will welcome them openly, adding chairs for them when they choose to embrace their practice. Sometimes I find my daughter just sitting in the room. She says that it just "feels so good" in there. She's right; that one room of my house seems to be full of magic and serenity.

Creating your sacred space will motivate you to sit in your chair every day. Make your space a place of love and healing. Here are some ideas for your room:

- Buy a comfortable meditation chair with lower back support or simply move a comfortable chair that you already own into the room.
- Buy a dedicated yoga mat and props for the room. Blocks, straps, bolsters, and blankets are nice to have.
- If you are transforming a guest room or your bedroom, consider covering the bed in a Zen-like fabric. Think natural prints and soothing colors.

- Place an altar near your chair. This can be any table, but it's nice if the height of it matches the chair height.
- Pick a scent. I love jasmine, but gardenia, lavender, and sandalwood are also excellent for relaxation. Place candles and incense on your altar and around your room.
- On your altar, place pictures of family and friends that you love. Include a picture of yourself from childhood.
- As your spiritual self grows, you might find that you want to place statues of Buddha, Shiva, Jesus, or other inspirational icons on your altar.
- Plan on storage for books and journals. Keep them nearby to inspire you before and after your meditation. Keep a journal in your space to record meditative experiences and thoughts.
- If you have a partner, it can be very powerful to meditate together. You may consider planning a sacred sanctuary for two. You may wish to include a massage table in your room.

OM Work, Week 1: The Good, the Bad, and the Ugly

An Exercise in Understanding and Forgiveness

"To understand everything is to forgive everything"

~ *Buddha*

My desk at the yoga studio sits under the stairs. My yogis practice yoga above me and pause at the cubbies outside of the yoga room to put their shoes back on and gather their things. They talk to each other up there, unaware of my presence. I can't help but listen and am always amazed by the things that come up after their yoga practice.

A while ago, I was sitting below and overheard one yogi talking passionately about how mean her mother was growing up. Her voice was bitter and hurt. Her mother had criticized her for her entire life. Her mother told her that she was skinny, clumsy, and lazy. This yogi has tried her entire life to please her mother, but all she gets in return is her mother's disapproval. She hears in her head her mother telling her how selfish she is. Because of that voice, she feels selfish and doesn't take time to nourish herself. Even her yoga practice makes her feel guilty.

She went on to say that the day she found out she was having a baby she swore to God she would never treat her kids the way she was treated. Instead, she makes a practice of telling her children that they are beautiful and kind. When they break things, she's quick to tell them, "It's okay, it was just a thing." She's quick with hugs and laughter.

I thought to myself how lucky she was to grow up with such a mean mom. I wondered what kind of work her children would eventually do and how they would serve the planet knowing how special they are. I wondered at the life her mother must have led to be so bitter and resentful.

I felt sorry for the yogi and for her mother. I prayed that she could forgive her mother and see the underlying blessing of the hidden gift her mother had given her. Her mother had given her the power to be a beautiful mom.

We have all been given hidden gifts through our suffering. The process of realizing the hidden gift ends the suffering. The following exercise, called "The Good, the Bad, and the Ugly," will allow you to unearth the hidden treasures in the less happy things you have experienced and also in the happy things. This exercise will take some time. Plan to work on it in bits and pieces. You may become very emotional during this exercise. Allow the emotions to come up, acknowledge them, and release them. Ponder and journal your thoughts.

Take a piece of paper and fold it into three equal sections. In the first section, write "The Good," in the second write "The Bad," and in the third write "The Ugly."

The Good

Write down three wonderful milestones in your life. These are accomplishments that you are immensely proud of achieving.

Examples:

I married the person of my dreams.

I put myself through college.

I was volunteer of the month at…

The Bad

Write down three not-so-wonderful milestones in your life that were the result of other people or outside situations. These are events or circumstances that changed the course of your life, and you are still unhappy about them.

Examples:

My dad left my family when I was a child and I never saw him again.

My mother abused alcohol and was mean to me.

I was fired from my job.

The Ugly

Write down three things you have personally done in your life that you still feel shame, disappointment, and/or grief over. Be honest and know that this exercise can be thrown away when you are done.

Examples:

I lost my virginity at age fourteen to a boy I hardly knew because my friend pressured me.

I cheated on my spouse.

I have unmanageable credit card debt and am not meeting my saving goals.

Now, for each item category, either just think about or, better yet, journal about the situation.

For example, write about where you met the person you married—what you have learned from this person, what you share, what values you have today because of this accomplishment. Writing about the good items can be pretty easy.

For the bad and the ugly, you need to journal around why the situation happened not just to you but to others who were involved. Think about the following questions and points:

- Who were the people involved?
- Why did they allow the situation to happen?
- What were they and/or you going through at the time?
- What were your thoughts?
- Walk in the other person's shoes.
- What did you learn?
- How did it change you?
- What was positive that came out of it?

In doing this, you will find compassion and forgiveness of the person, the situation, and yourself.

You will also realize that each of these life events happened for a reason. You did learn a lesson from them and you did grow in some way. Every single thing that has ever happened to you is perfect, because it got you to where you are today and today is perfect. When you can look at the good, the bad, and the ugly as gifts and be grateful, the suffering around the situation ends.

Week 2 Overview

Welcome to Week 2. I hope you had an enjoyable first week and spent time organizing and establishing your meditation practice. Week 2 gets a little more intense as we eliminate another one-third of our less-favorable habits and shift to two vegetarian meals per day.

This week, when you fill up your coffee or "other habit" mug, fill it all the way to the top and then pour off two-thirds of that cup. The same goes for any sweet treats and cheese. If you find you are really craving sweets, try the bliss ball recipe at the back of the book. Another great trick is to stuff a date with almond butter. It's super sweet and can curb those cravings.

You may find that your cravings begin to get the better of you this week. If this happens, consider making an appointment with an acupuncturist. He or she can place points in your ears to help you with cravings and even reduce stress levels. You may also find that you hit a wall this week with your cravings. You may start to have thoughts that you might be addicted to your habit. We will explore addiction and Ayurveda more deeply this week. Refer back to the section on dragons in Week 1 and start to ask yourself if you need to reach out during the Cleanse to begin the process of conquering that deep-seated habit or addiction.

Two vegetarian meals each day can be a challenge for some. I recommend that you make breakfast and dinner vegetarian. Meat should be consumed at lunch when your digestive fire is naturally at its highest. Notice that your digestion is strongest when the sun is at its peak in the sky at noon. Plan to look for vegetarian recipes in cookbooks and on the Internet. I highly encourage you to think of a meal that you love and figure out how to do a vegetarian version of that meal. For example, the steak and potato can become a portabella mushroom grilled with steak seasonings and a baked sweet potato.

You will need to explore the Cleansing Dish recipe found in the back of the book this week. I would love for you to practice many variations of this dish, including Beans for Breakfast. The final week of the Cleanse you will be eating an abundance of this dish, so you want to have many different variations or you will be bored with it. This dish is made from lentils. Unsoaked lentils cook in less than thirty minutes and are easy to digest. Know that the word *dahl* (or *dal*) is simply the Sanskrit word for "lentil." If you have access to an Indian grocery store or a store that stocks international products, you will find that dahl comes in many different colors. Buy all the colors and plan to experiment. Search the terms *dahl, dal,* and *kitchari* on the Internet and you will find thousands of recipes. Additional recipes can be found at **www.elementalom.com**.

You may not be used to eating beans. Because of this, you may experience gas, bloating, and irregular digestion. This week's discussion includes how to manage your changing digestion. Even if you are used to eating beans, you may experience dramatic changes in your patterns of elimination throughout the Cleanse. Many people fail to realize that their morning coffee, nightly glass of wine, and even dairy are stimulating elimination. Once you take these digestive crutches away, your body needs time to figure out its natural rhythm.

Included in this week's materials is a discussion of alternate nostril breathing. If you are finding it difficult to settle your mind for meditation, practice this before you sit to meditate. A little movement prior to meditation makes a positive difference in the receptivity and calmness of your mind. Consider practicing yoga for ten minutes or going for a walk to clear your mind prior to meditation.

Week 2 is a heavy week spiritually. You will work to cultivate the pure qualities of your soul, move away from the egoist reactions of your personality, and set intentions for the future. The intention-setting process, in particular, can be a little overwhelming to some. If you don't want to look at your whole life just now, go back to the assessment of your current situation that you completed before we began and simply intend for that one thing that you really wanted to shift. Do the entire intention setting process around that one thing.

Your meditation this week goes up to fifteen minutes each day. You will be bringing your soul qualities and your intentions into your practice. Your meditation now begins like this: ask yourself, "Who am I?" Repeat silently in your mind the characteristics from your Soul Profile (you will complete the profile later in this section). Read them to yourself if you need to. Next, ask yourself, "What do I want?" Read your intentions and desires to yourself (you will complete those later in this section as well). Then set it all aside and forget about it. Begin your meditation as directed in Week 1.

As The Earth begins to shift in your mind this week, you may begin to notice that accumulated clutter is starting to bother you. De-clutter one room of your house. It will feel liberating—you may feel lighter.

As the toxins begin to release this week, you may notice that you are feeling a little low on energy and even experiencing cold- or flu-like symptoms. You may experience acne. This is normal. Rest more and stay with the plan. Many who experience acne believe it is the sesame oil. It is not. Your skin is simply overloaded with the release that has already begun. It will clear.

Have an awesome week!

Week 2 at a Glance

For Your Body

Eliminate two-thirds of your less-favorable habits. This means when you look into your coffee cup this week, there is only one-third left.

Follow the Eating Routine

- Eat two vegetarian meals per day. If you are eating meat, eat it at lunch when your digestive fire is highest.
- Drink ginger tea throughout the day.
- Continue herbal therapy, one of each at morning and night.
- Continue daily self-massage.
- Continue daily movement—daily yoga and walking thirty minutes each day.

For Your Mind

- Meditate fifteen minutes each day. Use the mantra "so hum." Begin your meditation with your two questions: "Who am I?" and "What do I want?"
- Follow the daily routine.
- Schedule a professional Ayurvedic massage for Week 4. Look for a local spa that specializes in Abyangha.

For Your Spirit

- Practice daily silence. Drive in silence, cook in silence, and get ready for work in the morning in silence. Experience one hour of no talking each day.
- Spend some time in nature daily. This can be your thirty-minute walk.
- Each day, cultivate a sattvic soul quality and "move away from" an ego quality.
- Work every single day on your intentions and desires.
- Journal every day.

Other

- Make over your favorite dish into a vegetarian dish.
- De-clutter a room in your home. Clutter is a sign of an Earth imbalance in your mind.

Igniting your Digestive Fire or Agni: A Bonfire Lives in Your Belly

The purpose of the body portion of the Cleanse is to encourage your cells to release accumulated toxins into your digestive system and then to get them out of you in the traditional way. By that, I mean you eliminate them into the toilet. Your digestive system needs to be operating at maximum function to facilitate this elimination.

Imagine that you have a Fire in your belly. You do. In Ayurveda we call it *agni*. This Fire in your belly is just like a campfire. Imagine a campfire that is smoldering. Perhaps there are wet logs or leaves in it. You might grab the nicest piece of wood and throw it in the fire and it will not catch on fire. You digestion is just like that. I know so many people who are trying to lose weight by using techniques that logically should work. They eat a banana for breakfast, snack on carrots and celery, and then eat salads for lunch and dinner. They do not lose weight and become frustrated. How can this be? They are consuming all healthy food that are low in calories. They should lose weight, yet they don't. Why?

They don't lose weight for the simple reason that they have no Fire in their belly. They simply aren't able to digest even what appears to be a healthy food. Their bodies go into starvation mode. The undigested food sits in their digestive system and quickly turns to toxins. Furthermore, raw food is very hard to digest. It is cold, light, and dry. It aggravates The Wind element in your digestive system that is responsible for pushing food out. Many people end up constipated and bloated and have trouble sleeping when they eat raw foods.

Now consider the person who has a strong appetite, strong digestion, and strong elimination. That person can eat an entire pepperoni pizza with little effect. Keep in mind that if you consistently eat that way you put your strong Fire out, but every once in a while it's okay, and there will be few consequences if your Fire is strong. It goes in, it goes out. No problems.

That's the kind of digestive Fire you want to build. It goes in, it gets digested, and it goes out. It doesn't sit in your digestive tract full of bile and get reabsorbed by your very smart and efficient liver.

Week 2 of the Cleanse brings a lot of variability in your digestive system as your body attunes to the rhythms of nature. Your digestive system will undergo many changes during the Cleanse. You may find yourself constipated, regular, or going too much. This is your body adjusting to your new diet and re-establishing balance. Often, participants will think the herbs or the diet are interfering with digestion. Almost without exception, it's the elimination of the unfavorable habits that actually causes the imbalance. Many people unwittingly rely on their morning coffee or their nightly glass of wine to encourage elimination and regularity. (Both of these do stimulate the Fire in your belly).

Take the following steps to build your agni:

- Take your herbal supplements. All are meant to facilitate proper digestion. If you are constipated, double your dose of triphala.
- Follow the eating routine. Consistency teaches your body to attune.
- Replace butters, spreads, and margarine with ghee. Ghee is heating. In fact, you can melt a teaspoon of ghee into your warm milk substitute and drink before bedtime to facilitate elimination in the morning.
- Consider taking a few teaspoons of oil prior to bedtime. If you don't like the taste of sesame, use almond instead. It is much milder.
- Replace sugars and sweeteners with honey. Honey is heating to the digestion.
- Add spice to your food, such as peppers, black pepper, cardamom or cumin, cayenne, cinnamon, clove, ginger, turmeric, horseradish, and mustard.
- Drink hot water with ginger and lemon.
- Drink hot teas including Senna Tea. When choosing teas, always pick the pungent ones. Avoid words like *relaxing* and *calming*. The labels are usually red, orange, or yellow if they stimulate digestion. If you are constipated, drink a cup of senna tea.

- Take a pinch of ginger elixir fifteen minutes prior to eating.
- Habits like caffeine, alcohol, processed foods, and dairy affect digestion. Eliminate them and allow your body to make the natural adjustment.
- Eat a diet rich in pure foods. We discuss pure foods in the upcoming section called The Gunas.
- Cook all of your food and avoid raw foods.

A Special Note on Raw Food

I discourage you from eating raw food during the Cleanse. It is very hard to digest. If you must snack on veggies, blanch them first to begin the digestive process. Bring them to room temperature before you eat and then sprinkle with pepper and a little salt to facilitate digestion.

If you must eat salad, bring it to room temperature before eating. Put some Earth in that Windy salad by adding dried berries, nuts, and lots of olive oil or sesame oil to make your salad easier to digest.

Gas and Bloating: How to Minimize Your Suffering

We are not used to eating a lot of beans in our American diet. That means that we are going to have to get used to eating beans, and we will probably go through an adjustment that involves gas or bloating. Here are some tips to minimize discomfort during this period.

Cooking Your Beans

Preparing beans using the following tips will actually diminish the enzymes that cause gas and bloating:

- Soak your beans overnight
- Pour off the water that the beans were soaked in
- Rinse your beans before you cook them
- As the beans cook, skim off the froth and discard
- Add the following spices to your beans and your diet: cinnamon, fennel, dandelion, peppermint, turmeric, ginger, and lemon. All are used to treat gas and bloating.

You will likely suffer a little until your body adjusts. You will get used to digesting beans, legumes, and even the fiber of all the whole grains you are favoring. The following chart shows by body type the beans that are most easy to digest. Notice that if you are The Wind (Vata) body type, you are favoring the beans that cook in less than thirty minutes without soaking, including mung, dahl, lentils and split pea. That's because your digestion is delicate. You know if a bean can cook that quickly, it must be easier to digest. The Fire (Pitta) body type has very strong digestion naturally. You can eat the beans with the tougher skins like kidney beans and fava beans. The Earth

(Kapha) can have sluggish digestion. A few grains have been added for you to favor because they are complete proteins.

The Wind	The Fire	The Earth
lentils, dahl, mung	lentils, dahl, mung	lentils, dahl, mung
split peaT	split pea	split peas
tofu	black-eyed peas	lima beans
soy	black beans	quinoa
	chickpeas	chickpea
	All beans are good—	polenta
	have fun.	amaranth

All other beans are okay.

The Gunas

Sattva, Rajas, and Tamas

The gunas are one of my favorite concepts found in the Bhagavadgita and the practice of Ayurveda. The gunas represent three qualities of the mind that exist in all beings. They are depicted as chains binding us and attaching us to the world. They determine the way we behave and respond. The purpose of the gunas is to bind us through our sensory experience. We become attached to this physical world and to our egos if we do not free the binds of the gunas. Now, don't think these gunas are all bad. The guna known as sattva binds us to this world through happiness and the attainment of knowledge. That sounds pretty good to me.

In yoga, the gunas are depicted as part of the Kundalini awakening. The idea is that you have Kundalini (spiritual energy) located at the base of the spine. This Kundalini energy looks like a coiled snake in three coils. Each coil represents one guna. As you free yourself from attachment to the gunas, the coils unwind and the snake begins to climb up your spine and through your chakra system. The snake is feminine and represents your ego. The ego is aware that there is something much greater that is male that it wants to unite (yoga) with. This energy is the energy of Spirit. The snake climbs all the way to your crown chakra where the two unite and you become "enlightened."

Please don't get attached to the idea that you are awakening spiritual energy that has to go somewhere to unite with Spirit. You are Spirit, and you don't have anywhere to go or anything to attain. The psychology of Kundalini is to allow a process for self-study, better choice making, and right living so that you simply have a more peaceful, happy life that includes a tangible expression of spirit.

The first guna is called *sattva*. It means "pure." It is a state of consciousness established in peace, purity, truth, and light. Meditation, mindfulness, and the movement of yoga allow you to cultivate a sattvic mind. The spiritual exercises that you are participating in are allowing you to release the past that binds you, cultivate the pure qualities of your soul, diminish your ego reactions, and make nourishing choices. All this will lead to happiness. Ultimately we are to go beyond our sensory experience. Cultivating sattva is a good place to start. I don't know that anyone really knows what *going beyond* means anyway.

The foods that you eat are identified as a quality or guna that creates that quality in your mind and body. The gunas are (1) sattvic, meaning pure, (2) rajistic, meaning creating action, and (3) tamasic, meaning dull or dead. Just from that description alone, you would imagine that the sattvic or pure foods are far better for you than the tamasic or dead foods.

Sattvic foods make your mind clear and promote mental and physical peace. Yogis sustain on sattvic foods and avoid rajistic and tamasic foods. Sattvic foods are those foods considered to be first foods. In other words, these are all foods that humans have been eating since they appeared. Because they are the foods of our ancestors, they are part of our energetic expression and our bodies know exactly what to do with them.

The king of all sattvic food, believe it or not, is milk. There is a sacred place in Ayurveda for milk. This is not the milk that we know in the West, however. The cows of India are fed oils and herbs and are cloaked in garlands of flowers. The mothers feed their calves for two months prior to humans taking the milk. There are no hormones, antibiotics, or other artificial stimulants given to these cows. So, sadly, we must still avoid milk and use soy, almond, hazelnut, or rice milk instead.

The next most sattvic foods are honey, ghee, almonds, cinnamon, nutmeg, beans, legumes, vegetables, grains, fruit, all other nuts, seeds, and spices. These are listed in order of their purity. Make note that our Yogi Breakfast contains milk, honey, almonds, cinnamon, and nutmeg.

Rajistic foods are those foods that create action in your body. A little bit of rajistic is needed for digestion. Rajistic foods are any foods that are salty, sour, fermented, hot, or spicy. An easy way to identify rajistic foods is that they are usually an acquired taste: for example, coffee, alcohol, onions, garlic, hot peppers, citrus fruits, vinegars, and sour cream.

Some tomatoes are considered rajistic. Many tomatoes are raised to be sweet, however, and this offsets their heating nature. Eggs are deemed rajistic. I always remember that because any time my Fire son eats a hardboiled egg, he gets hiccups. The good news with the rajistic taste is that it is hard to over-consume. If you do over-consume, your body immediately responds with heat. You may experience a flash of heat in your body, indigestion, or heartburn.

Tamasic foods are deemed to be dead or dull. They create toxicity, or ama, in your body and mind. Ayurveda will tell you that all food that is processed, frozen, leftover, or microwaved is dead or dull. I don't agree. If you are buying organic processed food made the right way, you are fine. If you are freezing your leftovers appropriately with safety and care in mind, you are fine. Leftovers are timesavers, and we can safely store them. Leftovers that are more than three days old should not be eaten, however. I've done the research on microwaving, and it does not change the molecular structure of the food.

Most of the beliefs about tamas were developed long ago, before people were able to effectively store food. It was a safety measure. Microwaving did not exist five thousand years ago, so I don't really know who came up with the idea that it killed the food. While I agree that food that is cooked in the microwave does not taste as good, cooking it this way definitely does not change the food.

The following are some other foods that are deemed Tamasic:

Meat (regardless of whether or not it is organic)

Deep-fried foods

Stale or spoiled food

Garlic in excess

Alcohol in excess

Onions in excess

Soft drinks

Mushrooms (again, I think this was originally a safety issue—you pick the wrong mushroom, you die)

All things white, such as sugar, flours, rice, potatoes

Cheese (especially the hard cheeses)

Anything grown using chemical herbicides or pesticides or that has spent weeks on a truck getting to your grocery store

Oddly, really healthy and nutritious food if you overindulge in it

It is interesting to note that meat, cheese, and deep-fried foods are all full of saturated fat, which is known to cause heart disease and cancer.

During the Cleanse, you are moving away from these tamasic foods and learning to embrace sattvic (pure) foods. I make a game of going to the grocery store and checking out the carts in front of me in the checkout line. I estimate how much they have spent on food and nonfood. I also look in my cart and make sure that I have *only* food in it. I'm not saying you will never buy a bag of cookies again; just move your focus to spending your money on actual, pure food items.

How the Doshas Are Affected by Addiction

Week 2 can find you face to face with some of your deep-seated habits and addictions. You are intending to eliminate these, but you are struggling. Addiction comes in many forms: sugar, food, alcohol, sex, shopping, gambling, drugs, smoking, working, TV, and the Internet. Some people go in and out of their addictive behaviors easily. Some struggle an entire lifetime trying to destroy that dragon. There is a purpose to your addiction that you will only be able to see once you get to the other side.

Getting to the other side may be the hardest thing you will ever do. It takes acknowledgment of your helplessness, surrender, education, support, and sheer brute willpower.

This is how addiction works from an Ayurvedic perspective in body and mind. The energy of the addiction is the force of The Wind (Vata). The addiction initially creates an uplifting and euphoric feeling. The Wind begins to blow through your body and mind and you feel enthusiastic, creative, and wonderful. You have increased energy. However, the Wind tends to burn out quickly, so the feeling doesn't last. You have to consume/do more and more to continue to get that uplifting feeling.

Using or participating in the activity of our addiction gives our bodies the same reaction we get to the taste of sweet. The sweet taste, or the bodily reaction, makes us feel nourished and loved. A little bit of the sweet taste can make you feel safe, secure, and comforted. We naturally crave this sweet taste to balance and ground the energy of The Wind. The sweet taste is heavy and dense. It is found in comfort foods and the heavy American diet of meat, starches, and sugars. In excess, it causes you to gain weight and accumulate toxins and ultimately leads to diseases such as obesity, diabetes, heart disease, and depression.

Back to The Wind. You begin to crave the euphoric feeling, so you consume more and more of the source of the addiction. Finally The Wind energy gets extremely aggravated. Sleep patterns are disrupted, digestion becomes irregular, and shakiness may develop. You may become exaggerated in your speech, have an inability to focus or to concentrate, and be unable to listen to others. You may find yourself talking excessively and even rambling. Your dreams may become chaotic, and if you are deep into your addiction, you may experience a distorted sense of our shared reality.

Your life starts to go out of control, yet this dragon has you so firmly in its grasp that you can't even see that your life is out of control. In fact, you may feel that you are operating better than ever and think that you can take on more and more. Long-term thinking is impaired, and you begin to make spontaneous decisions that your deluded reality believes to be good. At this point, loved ones and friends may start to make comments about your behavior that don't seem significant to you or that you disagree with. You ignore their concern.

Over time, The Fire (Pitta) gets involved. You may begin to feel stressed, even when participating in the behavior you crave. The life you have created for yourself is becoming hard to manage. Perhaps you are grumpy and short-tempered with those around you. You start to feel that there is not enough time in each day to get everything done. You become resentful of the happy people floating around you in their stupendous states of bliss. In your mind they appear to be idiots without purpose. You believe that people don't understand you and aren't supportive of you. You become critical, judgmental, and controlling. You are living in fear, but you can't define the feeling as fear. It simply comes out as anger.

At this point, your health starts to really suffer. Your skin is ruddy. Perhaps you have acne breakouts, broken capillaries, redness, or irritation. Your eyes are bloodshot and glossy. You've put on some weight from your overindulgence or you are malnourished because your digestive Fire has been extinguished. Your blood pressure may go to a high level and you experience headaches, stressful sleepless nights, and upset acid belly. You are convinced that no one really loves you, and whether you will admit it or not, you are even more convinced that you are unlovable. You begin to alienate the people in your life, perhaps even eliminating them. You make really bad personal choices that may even put you in harm's way.

If The Fire doesn't completely burn you up, The Earth (Kapha) moves in. Now you feel completely miserable. You may be overweight. You are lethargic. You are depressed. You are full of despair and perhaps even suicidal. You now know without a doubt that no one loves you and that life is not worth living. You begin to accumulate clutter. You lay on the couch. Every movement seems like impossibility and you can't imagine a way out of your current situation. You are drowning and can't even muster the energy to raise your hand to greet any of the hands still being offered to you for support.

At this point, something needs to happen. Often this is the point where your addiction, that dragon living inside of you and controlling you, begins to fail. Now it doesn't even matter how much you consume/do, you never feel that sweet high from it. You never get a euphoric feeling.

Your health may completely give out. Your loved ones may abandon you. If you are lucky, you've hit rock bottom.

This is the turning point where most people will get down on their knees and plead for help. There is a divine spark inside of you, and it does not want to go out. It's a survivor. Rely on that spark to get you on and then off your knees.

Getting off Your Knees

This part is misery and bliss at the same time. You surrender. You know that you can't stay this way. You seek out help in the form of prayer, education, group therapy, or individual therapy. Now the real work of getting those elemental forces under control can begin.

Change is hard. However, you can transform a behavior in twenty-eight days, giving you an opportunity to fully recover from your addiction. Breaking an addictive behavior in twenty-eight days is not easy. Some people can do it without help, but most can't. Most people need support of others. The energy of the out-of-balance doshas is strong, and it takes time to bring them under control. While you are busy bringing them under control, they are fighting you as well as that dragon that doesn't want to lose its host.

Here is what happens to your elemental forces when you quit your addictions. All of the forces become simultaneously aggravated in an extreme way. You feel numb, super-stimulated, and out of your skin all at the same time. You sleep a deathlike sleep of exhaustion interrupted by insomnia. You crave sweet and are repulsed by its taste. You can't taste. Lights are too bright. People talk too loud. Silence destroys you. You worry; you stress. You are grumpy. You are overwhelmed by your emotions. You are excited and depressed.

Imagine an ocean experiencing a tropical storm. Imagine the force in that ocean creating those waves that are crashing onto the beach. The wave pulls out and then comes tearing back in. Now imagine you put up a wall about hundred yards from the beach. The wave continues to pull back, but when it comes crashing in, the wall stops it abruptly. The wave surges over the wall and then recedes, only to begin its approach again. In time, the wave adjusts, knowing that the wall is there, but initially, the wave is just as powerful and wants to take the wall out of its path. This is how the energy works in your body. The elemental forces are in full swing; they want to take out your wall.

The doshas will come back to balance in the same order that they went out. First Wind, then Fire, and then Earth. The Wind element will initially become very aggravated. Your thoughts will race and your cravings will make you feel insane. You will find you have excess nervous energy and nothing to do with it. You might shake and experience tremors. Sleep patterns are interrupted and you will become anxious and worried. You will crave sweets and salts. This is a critical time for distraction, rest, and support. If you are addicted to a substance, you will withdraw physically and mentally during this phase.

The Wind will begin to calm, and The Fire will move in. Now you will feel like taking some kind of monumental action. You may get angry with yourself, others, and your life in general. People will annoy you, causing you to become short-tempered. You may experience heart palpitations, sweating, and heat throughout your body. You may begin to feel empowered and this is when the idea of testing your new sense of strength may arise. You feel sure that you can have just one drink, one cigarette, one cookie, one shopping trip, and so on. But then you fail, and fail again, finally coming to terms with the fact that your source of addiction must be avoided at all costs.

The Fire begins to settle, and The Earth moves in. A "now what?" feeling settles over you. You've gone for some time without your dragon, and you begin to address the real dysfunction of your addiction. This is a boring time of hard work. You realize that you are just like everybody else. You realize that you've made a mess and that only hard work is going to get you out of the mess. You review your regrets and past mistakes. You get quiet. You spend time alone. You do intense soul searching and shifting.

You wake up and notice the birds are chirping with the energy of The Wind. You feel okay. Your first thought is not of your addiction, and you notice this. Your second thought is that your addiction actually served a purpose. Stay on the path.

Breathing Modalities for Meditation and Relaxation

Alternate Nostril Breathing

Alternate nostril breathing is a powerful way to balance the left and right sides of your brain. This pranayama will allow you to relax more quickly into your meditations, and it will help you focus, think, and sleep better.

You probably don't realize this, but you do not breathe equally through your left and right nostril. Depending on the time of day and your activity level, you favor one or the other. Your body automatically shifts from left to right every eighty minutes or so.

If you are breathing through the left side of your nose (Nadi Ida), the right side of your brain is activated. This is the side of your brain that doesn't understand boundaries, time, or individuality. It is your childlike and creative side. If you are breathing through the right side of your nose (Nadi Pingala), the left side of your brain is activated. The left side of your brain is the analytical planner that lives inside of you. It knows the past and the future, and it identifies with the "I am" part of us that believes only in separation.

To practice alternate nostril breathing, begin by gently closing your left nostril with your pinky finger or thumb (depending on which hand you are using) and breathing in through your right nostril. Then gently close your right nostril and exhale through the left one, and breathe back in through the left. Exhale through the right and breathe back in through the right. The idea is to take one full breath out and in on each side. You can stretch your breath to a count of four to six seconds, depending on your comfort level. Practice this breathing technique with your eyes closed.

Another Breathing Practice

Another amazing breathing technique that can be used to calm you and focus your mind is the dirga breath, three-part breath, or complete breath. This may be my favorite because it delivers exactly what you need regardless of the situation. If you are feeling anxious, stressed, or worried or you can't sleep, if you have a headache, or even if you need energy, this breath knows where to go.

To practice the complete breath, simply imagine that there is a balloon in your belly and fill the balloon all the way up with air. Then pull the air up into your lungs and exhale out through your shoulders in a slow and even manner. Don't be afraid to really puff your belly out as you take in air. You can do this sitting, standing, or lying down. Do it for a few minutes.

OM Work, Week 2: Ego, I'd Like You to Meet Soul

This is a quiz. From the left-hand column, circle six qualities that immediately turn you off. These are things that you really dislike in others. In the right-hand column, circle six qualities that resonate with you. Don't take too much time for this; just go with your gut. You may circle more or fewer if you like, but try to choose six qualities from each column.

Column 1	Column 2
Aggressive	Affectionate
Argumentative	Ambitious
Boastful	Ambitious
Changeable	Broadminded
Contradictory	Compassionate
Critical	Cooperative
Demanding	Dependable
Dependent	Diplomatic
Domineering	Efficient
Eccentric	Eloquent
Emotional	Enthusiastic
Headstrong	Friendly
Hypersensitive	Generous
Impatient	Helpful
Impersonal	Honest
Impressionable	Idealistic
Impulsive	Imaginative
Indecisive	Independent
Insincere	Inspirational
Intolerant	Intuitive
Irresponsible	Loyal
Lazy	Optimistic
Martyr	Original
Moody	Patient
Possessive	Perceptive
Quarrelsome	Practical

Rebellious	Protective
Resentful	Responsible
Restless	Self-sacrificig
Sarcastic	Sociable
Self-indulgent	Sympathetic
Self-pitying	Thrifty
Selfish	Unassuming
Sensitive	Versatile
Tactless	Witty
Two-faced	
Unpredictable	

Now that you have finished your quiz, take a look at the first column and then the second and say the following, "Ego, I'd like you to meet Soul." The first column represents your ego's nature. The second column represents your soul's nature. This is the idea of "mirroring." The things that you see in others that really turn you on or off are things that you yourself possess.

Now don't be too hard on yourself. If you had only circled qualities from the soul column and nothing from the ego column, you would be the most boring human walking the planet. Everything about you is perfect and wonderful, even what we perceive to be those not-so-favorable qualities.

"Everything that irritates us about others can lead us to an understanding of ourselves."

~ CARL JUNG

It's important to understand that you are not your body. You are not your mind. You are the embodiment of your soul. You are pure organized light. In the West, we have a view of our soul as being separate from our bodies. We see it as some other entity that is mysterious and far away in an abstract heaven. This is a perception or belief created by religious establishments, books, and media. The truth is that you are your soul. You are simply your soul covered in a sheath of humanity that we call ego.

When thinking of the ego, I like to think of the idea that when I incarnated to this world I walked through a sheet of plastic wrap. This plastic wrap molded all around my soul. The plastic wrap gave me the way I look, my mannerisms, and my preferences. It's my ego. It's very important. There is absolutely no way to get rid of that thing, regardless of what a lot of spiritual folks will tell you. What you can do, however, is learn to cultivate the more sattvic (pure) aspects of your ego. You can learn to respond rather than react from your ego.

For example, no one wants to be thought of as aggressive. It sounds negative. However, being aggressive is not really so bad. Being aggressive is a "large and in charge" ego quality that gets things done. If you think of aggressive as road rage, it sounds unacceptable, but if you think of aggressive as someone who has their mind set on a goal and is working hard to improve himself or herself or a situation, then it sounds pretty good. What you want to understand and learn to do is to accept the fact that you have an aggressive nature. You don't want to react aggressively with hostility or hate and run over people. You do, however, want to honor the fact that you can get things done with your determination in a kind way.

The soul qualities are easy to accept. Those are the characteristics we want to embrace. The hard part about those qualities is that we don't believe that we have those characteristics. I want you to convince yourself that you have those qualities and that you are absolutely wonderful.

This Week's Exercise

This week you are going to use the qualities you selected in the quiz as part of the exercise. You have selected six of each, so you have a set to work on for the next six days. You can rest on day seven. When you get up each morning, I want you to look at your list. Let's assume you picked aggressive from the left/ego column. In the morning, you will say, "I am moving away from aggression." Throughout your day, observe yourself and your environment. When you notice aggression in yourself or others, acknowledge it. Simply make the day a study of aggression. Be an observer with no judgment. Just notice.

That same morning, you will also pick a quality from the soul side of the quiz. Let's assume you picked the quality affectionate. I want you to make a mantra or affirmation from that quality. All day long, instead of having thoughts, I want you to think the phrase, "I am affectionate." Practice giving and receiving affection. Notice it in yourself and in your environment.

At the end of the day, journal around your experience, noting any synchronicities.

More OM Work, Week 2: Intentions and Desires

I equate happiness with the term *enlightened*. It is impossible to be happy if you are not getting what you want out of life. Most people don't get what they want out of life because (1) they don't know what they want, and (2) they haven't strategically planned. The purpose of the exercise below is to get you planning your life. Don't allow your life to happen. Plan it, direct it, and live it. Below are what I believe to be the foundations for a happy life. These are the areas of critical importance to achieving a feeling of success and wealth. The Cleanse has one major purpose: to get you happy.

It starts with the things that make you feel safe and secure (money) and moves to the things that make life worth living (relationships and Spirit). All are equally important and not one level can be sustainably fulfilling without the others also being in place.

Feel free to add and expand from here. I will discuss a directed approach for planning in all of these areas in the section called Intention Setting Process.

Goals for Your Physical Body

If you are not happy in your physical body because you don't like the way you look or feel, I can promise you that you will never be happy in life. It is imperative that you have optimal physical health and acceptance of your personal situation.

Make a plan for your physical body. Short term, you can plan to lose six to twelve pounds this month, release the accumulated toxic buildup of bad choices, and establish ease in your body through movement. Take your plan out further. Think about what you want to look like, taking into consideration your body type. If you are a Wind body, you will tend to be on the thin side and may never have the curves you crave. If you are The Earth, you will be curvy. Embrace your nature.

Your physical body's health really does point to how vibrant you feel. How do you want to feel when you wake up in the morning? What kinds of activities do you want to have energy for? Have you ever wanted to try skiing, belly dancing, or Tai Chi? Make your plan to participate.

Perhaps you simply want to rev up your love life. Do you find yourself too tired for love? Do you feel unattractive? Make a plan to bring some enthusiasm into this area of your life.

Refer to the "Ego, I'd Like You to Meet Soul" Exercise for This Exercise, "Goals for Your Ego"

For the rest of the Cleanse and your entire life, plan to work to cultivate the sattvic qualities of your soul and plan to learn ego responses versus reactions. Even though you only circled six this time, you can work your way through the whole list over time and touch on every aspect of a personality.

An ideal plan would include opportunities to help and serve that would actively help cultivate those qualities. Placing yourself in front of others who need compassion, love, and affection is the perfect way to make your soul shine. For those less-favorable qualities, plan to educate yourself. Get books, go to lectures, and find workshops or groups that can support you in taming the dragons of aggression, hostility, impatience, and control. Education is empowerment.

Material Reality: Areas of Your Life Related to Finances

This includes money and material possessions. To learn how to budget and how to get out of credit card debt, refer to the section called Financial Freedom or Money Moksha on page 123.

Retirement Goals

How old do you want to be when you retire? Do you want to work in a different field post-retirement? Will you stay in your current house? Do you have dreams to travel or obtain further education? What material items do you desire?

Home

Make plans for your home. What do you desire? Do you want to upsize/downsize? Would you like to live in a better neighborhood? Want carpet or new furniture? Need a new furnace or appliance?

Ability to Work: What Does Your Day Look Like?

Make a day-to-day plan that includes getting up, meditation, working, eating, playing, helping, serving, and sleeping. Write about your dream job, incorporating what you know of your dosha.

Professional Goals and Achievements

What is your dream job? How much money do you want to make? Are there honors and awards you would like to receive? What is your standing in your work community? How can you incorporate helping and serving into your job? (When you achieve this it this will make your whole life happier.)

Relationships: Your Personal Relationships with Others

This includes relatives, community, and neighbors. How often do you want to see your relatives? Plan one year out for all holidays. Where will you spend your holidays? How do you engage with your community and neighbors?

Partners

Stop, look, and listen. Assess your current partnerships. What are you lacking? What do you need? What are your partner's dreams, needs, and wishes?

Give what you wish to receive.

- Say thank you. Make it a daily practice to always say thank you to the ones you love for everything. This includes thanking for the small stuff and the big stuff.
- Honor when your partner is unhappy. Acknowledge that both you and your partner are going through transition. You can't solve another person's problems, but you can acknowledge that they are suffering with a simple hug and some kind attention.
- Ask for help when you are unhappy. Don't go it alone. Let your partner know what you are going through and how you intend to get through it. Tell them what you need for support.
- Daydream. Fantasize. Reconnect with your heart's desires for your relationships. Your dreams can come true.

Planning for Children

Do you want more? Are any moving out? Do you have grandchildren or are they on the way? What kind of role model do you want to be for your children?

Friends and Organizations

You *are* the people you surround yourself with. Plan to make new spiritually inspired friends who care about health, healing, and helping. If you are moving away from some less-favorable habits like drugs, alcohol, nicotine, and sugar, you need to intend to make a new set of friends, especially if any of these habits have become addictions.

Spirit: The Place Where It All Comes Together

Creativity: Pursuit of Your Personal Interests

Find a creative outlet. This is where your soul shines through. It doesn't matter if you dance, sing, write, paint, garden, decorate, cook, or play with crayons! Find something that is an outlet and do it every single day. The books you read, the music you listen to, the makeup you put on, and the clothes you wear all count as creative expressions. Enjoy all of it.

Spiritual and Other Study: Following Your Urges to Obtain Knowledge (Svadyaya or Self Study)

How will you maintain your spiritual and intellectual growth? Plan for workshops, events, religious affiliations and to get connected to a yoga community. FEED your soul.

Planning Your Death

Plan your death. Of course this sounds morbid, but we tend to have a lot of fear about death. Simply by planning to die at a ripe old age in your sleep after having the best life ever will start to calm those fears. If you have a deep-seated fear of death, read some books, watch some movies, and, best of all, volunteer to work with those who are passing. You will realize it's a beautiful process.

How Do You Speak With Spirit

How do you wish Spirit to communicate with you? God is always talking to you. Your mind has probably been too busy to listen or your mouth has been too busy talking to God to hear. You will start hearing now.

You will develop the ability to have all subtle body experiences as your mind calms and your meditation deepens. Plan to be in a tangible dialogue with God. A dialogue can be as simple as hearing the right message at the right time received through books, music, or friends. It can be as rich as dreaming of angels and meeting spirit guides. Some people see auras. Some people hear whispers in their ears. How do you wish to communicate?

Intention-Setting Process

It can seem daunting to sit down and think about what you want out of life. Perhaps you have never even considered it. You might find that your mind spins and it seems overwhelming. To assist you, I have prepared the following exercise. After you have done it once for just one of your desires, you will better understand the process. Use the categories above to inspire you.

Step 1

Write down your intention and desire in a positive way, comparing your present situation with your intention. Be honest with yourself about your present situation. Accept your situation as it is, accept responsibility for the situation, and intend to change it.

- What is your current situation?
- What are some choices you make every day that keep you stuck in this situation?
- What do you want your situation to be?
- What is your dream?
- What are you moving toward? Include your emotions about this answer. Give some details about your intentions and desires using all of your senses, including touch, taste, smell, sound, and sight.

Describe what it will be like when you attain your desire.

- Where will you be?
- What will you be doing?
- Who will be with you?
- What will you have?

Step 2

Now get more detailed. What steps to do you need to take to manifest your desire? Use your senses and envision the steps. Break down your intention and desire into small, concrete steps that are mapped out on a timeline that is reasonable and attainable. Be realistic.

Step 3

Now step back and look at the intention and desire from a worldview. These questions are not intended to discourage you from dreaming big. They serve as a reality check on how willing you are to shift your life. Sometimes we wish for things we are not ready for. Ask yourself these questions and notice how your body responds.

- Is your intention right for you?
- How is it going to affect your relationships?
- What will you have in the future that you do not have now?
- What are you willing to give up in order to attain your desire?
- Is your goal in alignment with your body, your mind, and your relationships?

Can you actualize your goal without outside assistance? You must be able to actualize your goals without the aid of others. For example, wanting to win the lottery is relying not on you, but on outside factors. *Earning* a million dollars is dependent on you. Meeting the love of your life while never intending to leave your home relies on outside interference because the love is going to have to knock on your door.

Step 4

Solidify your intention in a mission statement. Be very specific. For example: I will be building my eco dream home beginning in 2015 and moving into it in 2016. I will use the next three years to save, plan, and prepare for this transition, both personally and financially. My eco home will make me very happy and be a wonderful place to deepen my spiritual and familial relationships. (This is a desire of mine!)

Step 5

What do you need to manifest your intention and desire? Money? Education? If you are stumped here, find a role model. Do you know someone who has already achieved a similar goal? Model yourself after that person.

Step 6

What is one thing you can do starting this minute to move toward manifesting your intention and desire? Complete this sentence: Today, I will _____ to move toward realizing my dreams.

Financial Freedom or Money Moksha

In yoga, we use a term called *moksha*. Loosely translated, it means "freedom." This exercise is about finding financial moksha. So much of our stress and inability to manifest our intentions is because we do not have a healthy relationship with money. Some of this is due to a simple lack of understanding, because for many of us money, credit, and bills are confusing. Some of this is also due to a simple need to fill the void in our life with material items.

I will tell you that shopping and spending does buy temporary happiness. Who doesn't get a little lift from a new pair of shoes? Unfortunately, this lift is temporary. We continue to spend our way to happiness, and it's like chasing a 747 jet attached to a kite. Ultimately we are victims of the currents created by the 747's noxious fumes and mired in debt and even more unhappiness. It's time to take control, and to do that we must adhere to a budget.

Creating Your Budget

Do you know what you have? Follow this formula. Fill in the gaps and change as necessary for your own situation.

Begin with:

- Monthly net pay
  Make sure your employer is withholding your taxes, it's easier.

Subtract:

- Savings

  This equals 10 percent of monthly gross pay. That's the big number, not the net number above. You must do this to secure long-term happiness. Set up a separate bank account to transfer savings to.

- Mortgage or rent

  This includes insurance and property taxes. Have the bank hold these items in escrow. It's easier and stress-free.

- Utilities

  Electric, gas for home, trash service, water, homeowners association fees, etc.

- Cable television, Internet, home phone, security system
- Cell phone service
- Home maintenance

  Plan for your HVAC maintenance, gutter cleaning, lawn treatments, etc.

- Health insurance

  In a perfect world your employer is paying this and it's taken out of your paycheck. If not, call an agent and get some.

- Car payment
- Car maintenance
- Car insurance
- Groceries

  Allow $50/week per person in your home on average.

- Eating out

  Include your expensive lattes here.

- Children

  Lessons, sports, school fees, musical instrument rental, etc.

- Children's college fund
- Christmas (holiday) savings
- Birthdays and gift savings
- Other debt

  Add up monthly minimums on all. We'll address getting out of debt later.

- Pets

  Grooming, vet, feeding, etc.

- Entertainment
- Shopping

  Clothes, etc.

- Any other expense not on the list

After you have subtracted your expenses from your monthly net pay you will have a positive or negative number. A positive is positive cash flow. A negative is negative cash flow.

You might find at this point that you are (1) way over budget or (2) can't afford certain important budget items like college savings. Do not stress. This is a process, and this is where we begin. Start eliminating non-mandatory spending, starting with entertainment, shopping, and maintenance you can perform yourself. Is your car too expensive? Can you sell it and get a used car? Can you reduce your insurance, mortgage, Internet, TV, and cell phone plans by renegotiating?

You might find, too, that you don't know how much you spend. This is your time to start tracking your purchases. Start a spending journal. Keep it on the fridge so that the whole family can understand. No secrets. Put it out there; this is a team effort. What are you teaching your children by acting like everything is unlimited and okay? You are teaching them to overspend as adults. Get everyone on board. As you realize that you have habits and unrecorded expenditures, add them to your budget.

Special Note on Insurance

If you do not feel you can afford insurance, it is imperative to have "catastrophe" insurance at a minimum. In the event you incur huge bills, you are going to be taken care of; think car wreck or serious illness here. This type of insurance means that you have a large deductible; you are out-of-pocket on most care. Don't fret over that, because most doctors and dentists will help you with a payment plan. With the car insurance, it's not as easy, but it is required that you have car insurance.

Want and Need

During this Cleanse you are learning that material items are not fulfilling you. You've heard this before, but believing it takes time and can be hard to let go of. You are craving something more. Perhaps you don't realize it yet, but what you are craving is simplicity. Here are some things to do that can make you feel great about your choices, help the planet, and fill up some of your time if you had to cut your entertainment budget:

- Go through all your clothing. If you haven't worn it in the last two years, send it to charity or have a garage sale.
- Go through your pantry. Donate to the food bank all the unhealthy choices you have accumulated. I know! I know! I don't want the people dependent on the food bank unhealthy, it's just such a sad waste and they do need the calories.
- Go through your house. If your "stuff" has become a burden, start to eliminate. Give it away to those less fortunate. Donate. You'll feel great and free. If you need cash, have a garage sale or sell things on Craigslist.
- Plant a garden. This is going to cut down on your food budget and entertain you for hours on end. Your entire family can get involved in gardening. If you don't have a plot of land, use pots.
- Volunteer. We call this Karma yoga in the studio. Work trades and bargains with the people and places providing you services. You would be surprised at what small businesses are willing to do for you if you are willing to do for them.
- Buy bulk. Stop wasting your money on individually packaged items. Definitely do not buy water in bottles. Drink filtered tap water and fill up reusable bottles. Pack lunch for your entire family every day.

- Shop farmers markets and buy organic and local. Can you imagine the money that you can save by eliminating expensive items like meat, dairy, and processed food? Do you know how inexpensive beans, grains, and vegetables are? Feel like you are treating yourself to quality food and a few hours of entertainment by shopping the farmers markets, reading labels, and making educated choices.
- Kill the coupons. Unless you are getting a percentage off, they are never worth it. Most food coupons are for processed foods. Buy two cans of garbage and get one free. Cancel the newspaper that is sending you the coupons. News is free on the Internet.
- Buy used. Recycle, reuse, repurpose. What can you turn your old stuff into? What can you buy used? Flea markets and garage sales make great entertainment, too!
- Help and serve. Volunteer everywhere you go. You will find you have no time for TV, shopping, talking on your cell phone, and surfing the Internet. Your entertainment quotient will multiply. There's no better way to feel good about yourself than by giving. You will garner a whole new appreciation for the people and things in your life.
- Avoid. Don't go to the mall. Don't go to your fancy friend's fancy house. Don't look at the magazines that are trying to entice you. Don't covet. Don't be tempted. Withdraw your attention and you will find ease in your longing for possessions. Let *no* be your first word.
- Be strong. Tell people that you are on a budget…that you are sustaining the planet…that you are saving for your child's future. It will give them something to think about.

Get Out of Credit Card Debt

This is how you get out of debt. Cancel all but two credit cards. Keep the debit card. Don't charge another item. Pull your most recent statements and rank your cards by the smallest to largest amount owed. Fill in the following information for each card and repeat every single month:

- Card name or Bank of Unfulfilled Dreams (smallest balance card at top)
- Total balance
- Minimum payment
- Balance after minimum payment

Now that you know what you owe, pause and breathe. It's okay. We will get there. You aren't alone. The latest stats show that most American homes are carrying about sixteen thousand dollars in debt. Let's not continue to be *most,* though. Let's fix this.

Payment Plan

The credit card with the lowest balance is the one you are paying off first. Make all your minimum payments on all your cards listed and then give this card all the extra that you can. Then move to the next card after the first is paid off and cancelled. Don't use your credit cards anymore. You are done with overconsumption. Pause here to feel powerful.

Consolidation

Make an appointment with your bank. Take all of this information to them and tell them that you need help. If the first bank is not helpful, go to another. See what you can do to refinance your mortgage to the lowest rate and to consolidate your debt. Settle for nothing less than a fifteen or thirty-year mortgage. This is the job of the people who work for the bank. Let them guide you.

Always take advantage of the savings plans offered by your employer. They are the best out there and you won't get a better deal. If your employer does not offer a savings plan, go to that bank and ask them your options. Words like *Roth* will come up. Trust them. Do not feel embarrassed in any way if you are only able to save a very small amount to start. Start where you can and feel very proud of yourself for starting.

Set short-term goals for yourself, but think long term. Money doesn't cure all, but it makes life easier. It also allows you freedom from worry, stress, and desire. You deserve to have your heart's desires!

Plan to work on your intentions and desires for the remainder of the Cleanse. If you have not begun a journaling habit, this will get you to sit down and start writing. Good luck this week!

Week 3 Overview

Stay the Course

Congratulations and hugs to all! You made it through Week 2. Week 2 can be tough as we hit our walls with our habits and that monkey mind starts to get the best of us. I'm very happy for you that you are staying the course. If you find your resolve softening, seek solace in your yoga studio and pick up another inspiration book from the reading list to keep you motivated.

This week we eliminate that final one-third of your habits. Many people find that by Week 2 they give up most of their habits. If you haven't, this week is your week to conquer. When you fill up your coffee mug now, you go to the sink and pour it *all* out! You are free.

Because you have worked so hard to get rid of these habits, we want to spend some time this week talking about Karma and good choice-making. You are in a beautiful space right now, and all you have to do is continue to make good choices for yourself, for others and for the planet.

We will spend a bit of time exploring what I call sleeping dragons. These are your unconscious choice-makers or the bits of your personality that you are unaware of that are making choices for you. This is an important topic and goes to the heart of some of our biggest obstacles.

We will learn how your energy body is an extension of the entire universe and we will learn more about the chakra system and what chakras represent emotionally, physically, and spiritually. If you have been doing yoga, then you are probably hearing a lot about this at your yoga studio.

In Week 3 we are going to explore the Cleansing Diet that you will adhere to during Week 4. It will help you to get familiar with it now so that you can go grocery shopping and experiment with the Cleansing Dish. As discussed in Week 2, if you do not plan and prepare meals ahead of time you will become bored with your diet and derail yourself. Practice your dishes in advance and know that you can freeze portions to easily pull out for Week 4. If you plan and cook now, you can have a very simple kitchen-free week next week.

Week 3 includes some of the more esoteric features of the Cleanse, including the ingestion of ghee and sesame seed oil enemas. Go to the pharmacy and pick up three disposable small enemas. Don't freak out when you hear the work enema. This process is optional, but I would really like you to read the materials and consider it. The process is healing and is a great way to allow the toxicity to slide out of your cells and into your digestive tract. You should also practice making ghee. If you do not wish to make your own ghee, you can purchase it at www.elementalom.com.

At this point in the Cleanse, you may be experiencing symptoms of cleansing both mental and physical. This can be uncomfortable, but it is really good. As the body releases toxins stored deep in your cells, they enter your digestive system and are activated, causing you to feel physical symptoms such as fatigue, aches, pains, upset belly, and even flu-like symptoms.

Through meditation, your mind begins to release accumulated thoughts and memories. Additionally, the ego may begin to resist the spiritual transformation taking place, and you might find yourself wanting to overindulge or experiencing extremes of emotion. Stay the course. The following are some typical uncomfortable symptoms of cleansing:

PHYSICAL
Clogged sinus
Constipation
Cough
Diarrhea
Fatigue
Fever
Flu symptoms
Cold symptoms
Gas
Headache
Skin rash or acne
Stomach ache

MENTAL
Irritability and aggravation
Mild depression
Moodiness (extremes of sadness and happiness)
Impatience
Frustration
A feeling that your bones are too large for your skin (growing out of your skin)

This is part of the process. If you are having this experience, it's time to rest. Be gentle with your body and mind. Nourish yourself. This is a great time to receive a massage, take a day off, journal, and even nap! It's likely that you have been pushing yourself very hard for years and years. Let your body and mind heal. If your symptoms persist, something else may be going on. Do consult your doctor if symptoms persist.

Have a great week.

Week 3 at a Glance

For Your Body

- Eliminate the final one-third of your less-favorable habits. All habits are eliminated.
- Follow the eating routine.
- Eat three vegetarian meals each day.
- Drink ginger tea.
- Continue herbal therapy.
- Continue daily self-massage.
- Continue daily movement. Daily yoga and walking thirty minutes each day.

For Your Mind

- Daily meditation of twenty minutes. Use the mantra, "so hum." Begin your meditation with these questions: "Who am I?" "What do I want?" "How can I help and how can I serve?"
- Follow the daily routine.

For Your Spirit

- Daily silence. Drive in silence, cook in silence, and get ready for work in the morning in silence. Experience one hour of no talking each day.
- Spend some time in nature daily. This can be your thirty-minute walk.
- Complete your karma-busting exercise.
- Work every single day on your intentions and desires.
- Journal every day.

Other

- Practice making dahl. Make at least three variations. A sweet version for breakfast and two lunch and dinner versions.
- Practice making ghee. Use organic unsalted butter.
- Buy three small disposable enemas. Just buy the least expensive, as contents will be poured out and replaced with sesame oil.
- If you are ingesting ghee, begin on Day 19. Take 2 tablespoons on Day 19, 4 tablespoons on Day 20, and 6 tablespoons on Day 21. Begin enemas the evening of the final ghee ingestion.

Karma

Choose the Most Nourishing Choice

Karma is one of the most misunderstood of all Eastern thoughts. In the West, we view it as an endless cycle of suffering. What you sow, you reap. You get stuck in this process of doing things and getting things, and it never ever ends. It's frustrating because you believe yourself to be living a good life, and yet bad things continue to happen. Karma is perceived to be the chains that bind us. Ironically, however, Karma is actually your path to freedom. There are no chains. They don't exist. If you learn an appropriate method for making the best choices for yourself, your body, other people, and your planet, you will become a skilled choice-maker. Skilled choice-making makes no Karma.

Unskilled choice-making leads to unskilled action. This is Karma. Unskilled choice-making is making a choice based on ego-driven motives. When you choose out of doubt, fear, or personal motives, you create Karma. When you choose the most appropriate action, this is non-ego, skilled choice-making.

To cultivate skilled choice-making you will need to practice. The following is a list of questions you should ask yourself when making choices:

1. Is this choice easy to make?
2. Does it bring me happiness?
3. Does it bring the people around me happiness?
4. Does it make my body happy?
5. Does it make my planet happy?

You will know that you are mastering skilled choice-making when you have a sense that you are in the flow. When your choices become effortless, when you simply have a sense of knowing, then you are in that flow. This is where I can get a little esoteric and tell you that none of this is real. There is no time, there is no space, there is no body, there are no thoughts, and there isn't even pleasure or happiness. This is all just an illusion, and you are simply an expression of Spirit. You chose to come here to have this experience to clear all Karma so that you may melt back into Spirit.

What this means is that there is a plan for you that you initiated before you were aware of you. You are simply a feather blowing in the wind. When you accept that there is a wind blowing you, you learn to float upon it and go where it moves you. This is effortless choice-making. Things come up; you respond in a skillful fashion, and you keep moving.

This is the point where you ask: "Why do bad things happen to me now that I am a skilled choice-maker and choosing the best choices?" Things come up in this drama of life because you have had other lives that have generated Karma that you must clear up in this life. The self-realized guru (enlightened person) who develops cancer is clearing Karma from a past life. The sweet elderly person who is burglarized is clearing up past Karma. Conversely, the murderer who writes an award-winning novel from jail and receives national acclaim and monetary gain has brought in some good Karma from past lives.

The point is we are not to judge. We can't know. Most of us are walking around unaware of our past lives. That's why, when things come up, you turn yourself into a feather on the wind and simply go with it. Accept what comes your way. Fall back on your practice of skilled choice-making and deal with the issues as they come up.

Some serious issues will come up again and again. Typical Karmas we struggle with are addictions, bad relationships, self-doubt, and judgment. The exercise below will help you to identify your persistent, unresolved issues.

Karma-Busting Exercise

What is the one choice that you are making every day that is no longer serving you? This is your most undesirable behavior that you are actually aware of.

What is going to happen if you continue to make this choice? This is your cost/benefit analysis. What is it costing you? What is going to change in your life if you make a better choice?

Please write in twenty-five words or less what your new behavior looks like. Think of it as a personal mission statement to use as a guide. This is a positive goal. For example, if your sugar addiction is your negative choice, your mission statement could be, "I'm at my ideal body weight. My moods are even and positive. My skin is glowing. I have good relationships." This is called reframing the situation.

What must change in your life so that you make a better choice? This includes attitudes, perceptions, and behaviors. What can you do today to change your path in a positive way?

Follow-up

Was I successful? Why? Why not? If not, start over. Never stop working toward busting Karma. When you fall down, get back up. You are powerful when you fail and choose to start over.

Example of a Karma-Busting Exercise

Situation:	Choosing to stay up late every night.
Negative:	Continue to be tired, groggy, and uncreative and gain weight.
Positive:	I will be vibrant, clear, and alert with loads of energy.
Mission:	I jump out of bed with enthusiasm every morning!
Implementation:	I must honor that my body needs to rest to heal. I must place my body's needs above the needs of my family and my head.
Actions Step:	Get myself to bed. Talk to my spouse about my need to go to bed early and discuss a plan if my spouse doesn't want to change his/her routine.

Get my kids to bed on time so I can have a little relaxation and me time before bed. Stop obsessing over the cleanliness of my home. Just let it go a little bit.

Follow-up: Was I successful? I failed the first week, but I realized that stress and trying to relieve stress was a big factor in staying up. Watching a show or puttering around the house relaxes me. I'm now more focused on using my meditation, my breath, and mindfulness to eliminate some of the stress. I now look at bedtime as a reward for a hard day of work. It's a sacred time, and I did much better the second week.

The Sleeping Dragon

Unskilled choice-making includes unconscious choice-making, but I like to call it the sleeping dragon. These are decisions or choices that you make in total unawareness because, well, you aren't aware of them. These dragons drive your life and you must become aware of them to grow into a skilled choice maker. These are deep-seated Karmas. The only way to become aware of your unconscious choices is to start listening to the people around you. When someone tells you that you are a certain way, believe him or her. If it is something you hear a lot, really believe it. Now, I'm not talking about accepting into your heart every single criticism, but I would bet that the people closest to you have noticed certain repeat behavior that they express to you…especially your mother. This behavior may include any of the following examples:

- You are stubborn.
- You never change your mind.
- You always change your mind.
- You never commit to anything.
- You are a martyr.
- You are a victim.
- You never make a decision.
- You lack follow through.
- You are always late.
- You don't listen.
- You are critical, judgmental, or controlling.
- You are always so perfect.

This list is very simplistic, so I will give you a very personal example that goes very deep. This is a great example of how far you can take this process and the huge effects of your sleeping dragons. My sleeping dragon centered on relationships. My father abandoned my mother and me when I was thirteen. Since then, I have lost a lot of people in my life, including family, friends, and lovers. If you had asked me how I lost them, I would have told you that these people left me. I would have sounded hurt, betrayed, and bewildered.

Through self-study and sheer desperation to have any relationship last, I became aware of my sleeping dragon. I became aware that people don't leave me. I leave people. You see, my father choosing to leave me caused me great suffering that I could not effectively deal with as a child. Deep down inside of myself, this dragon decided to protect me. Rather than having people leave me, I would unconsciously choose to destroy my relationships, pushing people away so that I could choose the moment that they left. In doing that, I had control of the pain that I deemed to be inevitable. People don't leave me. I leave people. That was my hidden dragon.

I didn't know to look for the hidden until I became conscious of the idea that you can unconsciously choose. Once I became aware to look for the hidden, it became obvious. I knew where to look only because I looked to what is most painful and began to observe it…and me. This dragon is not dead, but it no longer makes choices for me. When I feel it rearing up in the form of insecurity, fear, and an insane desire to run away from my life, I look it straight in the eye. Sometimes, this means I have to ask for help from the people around me. I tell them I'm suffering, I feel out of control, and I need them to help me sit still because I'm scared of me.

A common sleeping dragon that I see over and over when teaching the Cleanse is codependency. If you grew up in a home where one or more parents were alcoholic, abusive, or abandoned you emotionally on any level, you probably have some deep- seated sleeping dragons to unearth. Let's discuss those next.

Common Sleeping Dragons
Samskaras Are Deep Impressions

We are all here on this earth to enjoy this big play and to learn lessons our soul wishes to master. In Sanskrit, this play is known as *lila.* Much goes into the path we take in life, including Karma from previous lives and Karma created in this life. These Karmas create impressions called samskaras. It's a scarring of your brain that creates a behavior loop you may be unaware of.

As humans, we share a common experience unique in that it is our own, similar depending on the country you are born to. Each of us, as unique as we are, are still molding our thoughts and choices in common archetypes or stereotypes. Some of this is good and some challenging.

Yoga includes a process of self-study. Through observation of your thoughts, words, and deeds, you can begin to identify your stereotypical patterns that are hidden in a belief system learned in childhood from parents and society. You become the observer disconnected from that being observed. You simply observe your thoughts. The distance created gives you space and time to make other thoughts and ultimately choices. A good practice for self-study is not only to gather information and education, but also to ask yourself the following questions when observing your thoughts:

- Why am I thinking what I'm thinking?
- Is the voice in my head my own or someone else?
- Why do I believe what I believe and others do not?
- Am I making the same choices that my parents made?

Some stereotypes that are prevalent in our American culture are the codependent and the addict. Answer a few of the questions below and see if you fall into any of these stereotypes. Don't feel bad if you do. Just begin the process of learning about yourself and cultivate a plan to break the mold. These are some of our most common sleeping dragons.

Are You Codependent?

- Do you suffer greatly from saying no?
- Do you put yourself in situations where you really didn't want to be, but commit anyway? Do you find yourself resentful in these situations?
- Does helping others make you feel worthy or superior?
- If you stopped helping, would you feel guilty or worthless?
- Do your relationships end when there is no longer a need for your help?
- Do you resent those you help and think that they are not grateful?
- Do you have a very hard time asking for help and rarely do?
- Do you have a hard time receiving help?
- Do you pretend that everything is fine?
- Do you surround yourself with people who live in chaos and have one problem after another?
- Did you grow up in a family that had a lot of emotional chaos or addiction problems?
- Are you emotionally involved with an addict?
- As a child, did you take on the role of holding your family together?
- As an adult, is it important for you to be thought of as the dependable one?
- Are you a negative person?

If you answered yes to any of these questions, you may be what is termed codependent. Your mind has simply wandered into the territory of this archetype or stereotype as a means of coping. It's an unhealthy pattern that you can and must break to achieve happiness. To break the habit, simply notice your thoughts. When you experience thoughts that resonate with the list above, take a pause. Tell yourself you don't have to think that way or be that way. Immediately replace the negative or less-favorable thought or belief with an affirmation. A great affirmation for codependents is "my best is good enough." I love to think simple affirmations like "I am light," "I am love," "I am joy," "I am a divine expression of spirit," and "I am a thought of God." This practice will take three months and even beyond a year to really create the grooves and awareness in your brain to automatically shift to the new thought pattern.

Are You an Alcoholic?

Defining an alcoholism is much harder. It can take up to sixty years for the habit of drinking to turn into alcoholism. Many people will binge drink for a few years while they are going through life transition and then get it under control. Many people simply limit their drinking to the weekends. It is unclear. If you search the Internet, you will find many quizzes that you can take to do a self-assessment. I don't really love any one in particular because of the grey area around alcohol. I personally believe that substance abuse is when you consume to relieve or escape your problems, not realizing that the substance is creating those problems.

At this point in the Cleanse, if you are craving alcohol and your mind continues to wander back to thoughts around drinking, then I suggest you empower yourself with education and sit down with someone for a one-on-one session. It would be super hard to do, I know, but to simply ask your family if they think you drink too much is powerful.

Are You Addicted to Sugar?

- Do you eat refined sugar every day?
- Do you find it hard to go a day without sugar?
- Do you crave sugar, coffee, chocolate, or alcohol?
- Do you hide sweet snacks in your home or office?
- Do you have a hard time stopping consumption after a small serving of sugar?
- Do you have very few periods of time without sugar in your house?
- Do you find it hard to resist sweets if they are in your home, office, or at an event?
- If you skip sugar, do you experience shakiness, fatigue, or altered mood (negative mood)?
- Do you eat something sweet after every meal?
- Do you start your day with coffee and a sweet treat?
- Do you drink sweetened soft drinks on a daily basis?

If you are suffering from a sugar addiction, group therapy and the support of a counselor is the recommended course. Find a group that resonates with you on a spiritual level. The choices you make unaware can shape your whole life. They affect your health, your family, your relationships, and your job. Begin this process now.

Your Energy System
The Chakras (Chakra Translates to "Wheel")

In yoga, Ayurveda, and most Eastern traditions, the body is diagnosed and treated as an energy system. The diagnostic tool most commonly utilized is the chakras. You are more than your physical body. You are a vibrating creature that vibrates in a certain pattern that is associated with frequency, sound, and color. You are a rainbow of seven chakras seated on your spine.

Depending on what you study, you will learn that there may be more than seven chakras. There are thousands of nadis and even more meridians where the vibrations cross paths. In yoga, we work with 108 total channels. All of these in attunement create a healthy body and mind. The chakra system also offers a way to explain how your mental status affects your body. Each chakra sits on a gland of the endocrine system.

In yoga we practice certain poses that stimulate your glands. During the pose we will often tell you to place your attention on a certain chakra and invite in a corresponding emotion. In science we know that blood flows where your attention goes. In yoga we believe that subtle energy also goes where you place your attention and a healing occurs. This is why yoga makes you feel so good.

There is a practice called toning. The key of the chakra is sung using the following sounds (lam, vam, ram, yum, hum, sham, and om) with focused attention on each chakra. You can bring color into the visualization. You can participate in drumming, singing bowls, and other fun ways of bringing sound into your practice. Below is a discussion of the seven chakras.

The Root Chakra (located at the base of the spine)

Muladara translates to "root support." Energetically it is a very earthy chakra. It resonates with the senses of smell. Spiritually it represents your everyday actions and choices. Your Karma lives in this chakra. The foundation for all of yoga is called *ahimsa,* which translates to "nonviolence." A strong foundation for a happy life is built from nonviolence in thoughts, words, and deeds. Taking yourself and others into consideration and always choosing the most nourishing choice for all will guarantee that you have a good foundation for a happy life.

Fun Facts About the Root Chakra

Gem Therapy: garnet, ruby, bloodstone, red jasper, smoky quartz, black tourmaline (my favorite)
Oil Therapy: clove, cedar, sandalwood, pine
Mantra to tone into the chakra in the key of C is lam.

The Sacral Chakra (located just below the naval)

Svadhisthana is the seat of your vital energy. It's where the earthy nature of the root chakra merges with the watery nature of the sacral chakra. Often the two are depicted as merged. It resonates with the sense of taste. It's where you begin to interact with others in the desire to create. Creation takes place when you are tapped into the effortless ease of the universe. There is a stream of consciousness that you are floating in. You struggle when you try to swim out of that stream or swim in the opposite way. Simply allow yourself to go with the flow and stop struggling in your life. Find a creative outlet. When you are in the moment of creation, your soul is shining through.

Fun Facts About the Sacral Chakra

Gem Therapy: ruby, carnelian, citrine
Oil Therapy: sandalwood, jasmine, ylang ylang
Mantra to tone into the sacral chakra in the key of D is vam.

The Solar Chakra (located just above the naval)

Manipura translates to "city of jewels." It is the place in your body where you put your dreams into action. The heart is your real dreamer, but without action, your dreams will not come to fruition. This is a fire chakra and represents the rajistic quality of taking action. It resonates with the sense of sight and with your soul qualities. As you practice affirmations of your soul to develop your sattvic qualities, imagine that you are seeding them in this chakra. Do your work of setting your intentions for your life.

Fun Facts About the Solar Chakra

Gem Therapy: gold, topaz, amber, citrine
Oil Therapy: chamomile, lavender, rosemary, peppermint
Mantra to tone into the solar chakra in the key of E is ram.

The Heart Chakra (located at the sternum)

Anahata translates to "unstruck." It's an amazing concept. Something that is unstruck makes no sound. No sound is the center of everything. Many yogis believe that your heart chakra is the center of your existence.

If you look at the yantra (the picture on the chakra) you will see one triangle pointing up and another pointing down. They are superimposed on each other and surrounded by a circle. The two triangles joined create the Star of David, a Kabalistic symbol as well as a yogi symbol. The triangle pointing up represents the masculine. The triangle pointing down represents the feminine. It is the union of opposites: male and female, giving and receiving, hot and cold, solar and lunar. The enclosing circle represents Spirit.

This is the symbol of Hatha yoga. It is the yoking of opposites in body and mind encased in spirit. It's quite beautiful. Simply practicing understanding, compassion, love, giving, and receiving will allow your heart to flower. If the heart is flowing, all the other chakras flow, too.

A fun meditation to practice after Shavasana is to come to a seated position, roll your head down so your chin is reaching toward your heart, and envision yourself sitting in this yantra. Your head is at the top of the first triangle. Your bottom builds the base. Just sit there—no mantra, no thought—and enjoy.

It is interesting that the heart chakra resonates with the sense of touch and is the center of giving and receiving.

Fun Facts About the Heart Chakra

Gem Therapy: quartz, rose, rhodochrosite, jade, chrysoprase, emerald
Oil Therapy: lavender, jasmine
Mantra to tone into the heart chakra in the key of F is yum.

The Throat Chakra (located at the throat)

Vishuddha means "purity" or "purification." This chakra resonates with the element space and the sense of hearing. It is thought to allow people to speak their truth. Speaking your truth means knowing your truth. I can only give an esoteric discourse on this chakra because to really understand it you would have to understand and accept detachment. You must have the experience to understand. The truth is that you have everything you need. There is no need for seeking and searching. It is all right here.

A practice for understanding this is to simply surrender to Spirit. In the midst of the chaos, throw your hands up and trust that you are supported.

Cultivating healthy detachment from people and things is part of the process. It's not hard to figure out what you are attached to. Think of the people, things, and situations in your life that you obsess over, worry about, and try to control. Now think of the people, things, and situations that are not present on your mind other than to occasionally wander to it or them. That's attachment and detachment.

Fun Facts About the Throat Chakra

Gem Therapy: turquoise, kayanite, sodalite, blue agate, lapis, amazonite, larimar
Oil Therapy: frankincense, sage, eucalyptus
Mantra to tone into the throat chakra in the key of G is hum.

The Brow Chakra (located between the eyes at the brow)

The *Ajna* chakra is the seat of your soul. Many believe it is the residence of your soul. Your intuition develops here. Your soul does not experience time or space. Your soul has access to all that has been, all that is, and all that will be. When you connect with your soul through meditation, mindfulness, and silence, you gain access to this realm. That is why you can develop a sense of knowingness or psychic abilities.

The brow chakra is known as Ajna. It is located just between your eyes, on your pituitary gland, the master gland controlling all the others. It resonates the color indigo like the night sky and makes the sound of A on a musical scale.

The brow chakra is where your intuition lives. The lesson is to simply trust yourself. Many yogis believe that your soul resides in this chakra.

Fun Facts About the Brow Chakra

Gem Therapy: angelite, amethyst, sodalite, celestite, phenacite (use phenacite with caution, as it can cause headaches)
Oil Therapy: jasmine and peppermint
Mantra to tone into the brow chakra in the key of A is sham.

The Crown Chakra (located at the top of the head)

Sahaswara means "complete within oneself." A thousand-petal lotus represents it. The most powerful and effective way to connect to Spirit is through silence, observation of your thoughts, prayer, and meditation. Each person has a unique experience of Spirit. It is said that if there are seven billion people walking the earth, there are seven billion ways to heaven.

When establishing your relationship with Spirit, use what you know and what is familiar to you. For example, many Americans coming to yoga and learning about meditation will begin to bring Buddha, Krishna, and Hindu deities like Genesha into their practice through mantra and visualization. This can be very difficult if you do not have an experience of those religions. It's like trying to describe what a rose smells like having never smelled one. Use what you know. Use your foundation, whatever it may be. Know that you don't have to be religious to be spiritual.

Explore all the masters. There is much to learn from all cultures and traditions, but make your personal practice what deeply resonates with you.

Fun Facts About the Crown Chakra

Gem Therapy: selenite, quartz, amethyst, celestite, phenacite (use phenacite with caution, as it can cause headaches)
Oil Therapy: vanilla, jasmine, rose, lotus
Mantra to tone into the crown chakra in the key of B is om.

Dharma

Dharma is a Sanskrit word that is commonly understood to mean "life purpose." Dharma, however, has a much deeper meaning than simply your life's purpose. Dharma is "that which you must uphold." It is a contract that your soul signed prior to incarnation into this life. You have agreed to live a certain type of life, experience specific things, and ultimately be of service to your fellow humans.

Let's imagine that you don't believe in reincarnation. Many people don't. If that is the case, dharma is about being on your deathbed and looking back at your life knowing that you had a great life. You want to leave this world thinking, "Wow, I rocked it!"

When I teach The Elemental Cleanse in person, I always pause to ask the participants if they know what their life's purpose is. Almost without exception, no one raises a hand. I think this is for several reasons. First, our culture does not stress that we are here for a reason, and second, our culture does not stress service. Most people have never even paused to consider that there is a reason for being on this planet.

Ask yourself the following questions:

- Why am I here?
- What is my life's purpose?
- How can I be of greater service to others?
- What do I naturally do well and love that I can offer to the world?

If you find that you have no answers to these questions, I want you to begin the process of uncovering your life's purpose. Think of it as solving a puzzle. First, accept that you are here for a reason and that reason does include service to humanity. Now begin a list of things that you naturally do well.

Examples include:

- I love the energy of children.
- I find the elderly fascinating and love to listen to their stories.
- I love to negotiate.
- I feel at home on the stage and love being in front of people.
- I love to talk to people and help them solve their problems.
- I love to cook, to read, to write, to dance or to sing.
- I love managing the finances of my home or work.
- I love creating.
- I love planning.
- I love animals.
- I love technology.

Chances are that one of those sentences resonated with you. That means that it is part of your purpose. Notice that I said *part*. Your life purpose is a blend of your passions. For example, if you love the energy of children, chances are pretty good that you would enjoy being a parent. It's possible that you would even enjoy teaching or taking care of children in a day care setting, but maybe not. Raising your own children would certainly be part of your purpose, while raising other children may not be.

If you love to negotiate, wouldn't it be fun to be a lawyer or a salesperson? If you love standing up in front of people, perhaps you would like a job that includes public speaking or even acting. If you are great at math, perhaps you would enjoy being an accountant, a math teacher, or an engineer.

Use your gifts and the ease or grace in your body and mind to your advantage. I find it interesting that so many people choose experiences based on other peoples' expectations. I often meet talented visionaries and artists who ended up becoming doctors, lawyers, and engineers because of a parent's expectation. I also meet many parents who had children at the request of a spouse; they really suffer as parents. It's hard work for them. If you don't love something, don't do it. If you do love something, you are supposed to express that gift. This is the grace in your life. Let it flow.

Many people begin the process of connecting to their purpose full of criticism for self. When you look at the archetypes of our society, you may feel intimidated or less than another. Some people have a very dramatic life purpose. For example, there will only be one first black president of the United States. That purpose is taken. There will only be one Mother Teresa, one Gandhi, and one Martin Luther King, Jr. They had some pretty big purposes and are archetypes for the rest of us to aspire to. They are the heroes that motivate us on our personal journey.

Most people have a very simple purpose, and it is at the root of their happiness. If I were to question the seven billion people currently residing on this planet about their happiness and what they desire, most would answer the same way. All people collectively want love of another, comfort of family, health, and a job that they find rewarding. What this means is that most people are simply here to have a rather simple and lovely life.

I was speaking to the woman who delivers the mail to my studio the other day. She told me that she loves her job. She gets to walk every single day and loves the outdoors. She meets lots of people and loves knowing all the shop owners. She enjoys the security and benefits of her job with the postal service. She is certainly serving humanity because she is bringing the mail every day. She's in her dharma. She has combined her love of exercise, nature, and socializing in the perfect way for her.

Many women taking the Cleanse are stay-at-home moms. I see a trend among stay-at-home moms that they feel they are missing something and not meeting expectations. Most have gone to college and worked prior to having children. Their education and jobs were a huge source of esteem. Because our society expects all things from women, including working, paying the bills, having children, raising children, and taking care of the home, women are conflicted. It is important to understand that there is no bigger purpose than raising children and teaching them to be sattvic and of service. You will go back to work when the time is right. For now, enjoy your life and put your energy into your children. You are in your dharma.

During Week 3, I want you to begin the process of thinking about your purpose. Do the exercise above. In addition to that, I want you to start looking for ways to be of service in your life. Be the person who gets doors for others, cleans the kitchen, and changes the roll of toilet paper. Start small and you will be surprised as opportunities to serve pour in.

We are going to bring this OM work into our meditation this week. When you sit for meditation, begin with your questions:

1. Who am I? Use the answers from "Ego, I'd Like You to Meet Soul" to answer.
2. What do I want? Use the answers from your intention-setting process.
3. How can I help? How can I serve? Don't answer these questions. Just throw them out to the universe and see what comes your way.

Do let all of these thoughts go and begin your mantra meditation.

Cleansing Diet

This is your diet the final week of the Cleanse. Practice your dishes during Week 3 so that you are satisfied and like your food for Week 4.

The Cleansing Diet is very simple. It is wonderful to make your dishes in advance of Week 4 because they freeze easily. If you plan well, you can have a cooking free week the final week of the Cleanse. Look for recipes at www.elementalom.com and at the end of the book.

Plan in Week 3 to organize the following for Week 4:

- Any bean that cooks in less than thirty minutes without soaking, including dahl, dal, lentils, split peas, kitchari
- White or brown rice, because they are easy to digest
- Steamed vegetables or vegetables cooked into dahl dish
- Bliss Balls if you need to snack on something sweet
- Ginger tea
- Ginger elixir before meals
- Yogi Breakfast

The Elemental Cleanse is founded in the traditions of Ayurveda. Specifically, the Cleanse is a modified self-administered purva and pancha karma. The purva karma experience is the first three weeks of the Cleanse. This process allows your mind and body to prepare to receive the final week of the Cleanse or pancha karma. The Cleanse has been modified to some extent from the Eastern traditions because some of these traditions simply would not resonate with our Western culture. Further, the emotional and spiritual exercises have been developed with our culture in mind.

What Is Panchakarma?

Panchakarma is a methodology used in India to flush out toxins within the mind, body, and emotions. It is a powerful way to connect or reconnect to spirit. It is typically undertaken with the changing of the seasons or when disease is in the body. It cleanses the body, improves digestion, improves metabolism, and reestablishes life purpose and connection to Spirit. It should be performed, at a minimum, once a year by all people. If you are suffering a serious illness, depression, or weight gain, it should be performed with your course of treatment, or ideally before, so that your body can receive treatment and process efficiently.

In India, panchakarma consists of oleation (ingesting oil through nose, enemas, eating, and skin) laxatives, heat therapy, vomiting, and bloodletting. In a self-administered panchakarma, you do not participate in vomiting and bloodletting, as an Ayurvedic physician with a medical degree must guide this. Both practices can be dangerous if performed without supervision.

Panchakarma works on the dhatus or tissue layers in the following ways:

- The immune system is flushed (rasa, or lymphatic fluid and plasma). This improves immunity and the body's ability to fight disease. Emotionally, rasa is associated with the ability to feel joyous. Rasa is thought to be a sacred fluid that sustains life.
- The blood (rakta) is purified. Emotionally, rakta is associated with the ability to live passionately and to have vigor.
- The skin and muscle (mamsa) release toxins. Emotionally, mamsa is associated with the ability to discern in any situation.
- The fat (medas) is flushed. Medas is associated with feeling lovable and giving love.
- The bone (ashti) is rejuvenated. Emotionally, this will give you confidence and clarity of intention.
- The nervous system (majja) is soothed. This gives calmness and clarity.
- The reproductive tissues and fluids (shukra) are restored, giving creativity.

It becomes obvious from the above discussion that your physical and emotional bodies are not separated. The flushing of ama is on all levels.

Ghee and Enemas

Part of the Cleanse includes a couple of things may seem rather odd. The first is the ingestion of ghee. Ghee is clarified butter. In small amounts no larger than one teaspoon at a time, ghee is heating and stimulates digestion. If you are constipated, you can actually heat a little milk, add a teaspoon of ghee to melt, and drink to facilitate elimination. We ingest ghee prior to our final intensive week to loosen up the final bit of ama (toxins) that have been brought to the surface dhatus by the three initial weeks of good living and eating. The ghee also pacifies The Wind (Vata), cools The Fire (Pitta), and nourishes The Earth (Kapha). The ghee, in combination with the ginger tea and the extra cumin and turmeric added through our Cleansing Dish (kitcheri) cause the cells to spit out the toxins. Finally, the small intestine is flushed with oil and all the loosened toxins come out. You then go into the final phase of eating easily digested food and then rebuilding agni (fire) by eating for your dosha.

"Ghee is sweet in taste and cooling in energy, rejuvenating, good for the eyes and vision, kindles digestion, bestows luster and beauty, enhances memory and stamina, increases intellect, promotes longevity, is an aphrodisiac and protects the body from various diseases."(Bhavaprakasha 6.18.1)

Optional Ghee

If you wish to rest your digestion and oleate your body prior to Day 22, which begins the final flush from your system, then take the following steps. On Day 19 (during Week 3), ingest two tablespoons of ghee gradually throughout your meals. Melt and drizzle over veggies. Notice how you feel. If you feel queasy or if you lose your appetite, you are done. Have an oil enema that night and start the Cleansing Diet on Day 20.

If not, on Day 20, ingest four tablespoons of ghee. Notice how you feel. If you feel queasy or if you lose your appetite, you are done. Have an oil enema that night and start the Cleansing Diet on Day 21.

On Day 21, ingest six tablespoons of ghee. Regardless how you feel at this point, this is the maximum amount of ghee recommended, so have an oil enema that night and start the Cleansing Diet on Day 22.

Optional Enemas

The enemas either start on the evening of Day 22 (if you are not taking ghee) or on the night that you lose your appetite if you are taking the ghee. Do one each night for three nights in a row. Follow the enema package instructions, but remember to dump out their product and fill up with the sesame oil that came in your cleansing kit if you purchased one. If you did not purchase a cleansing kit, you will need to buy organic sesame oil.

The key word here is *optional*. You will still have a great experience without the ghee and enemas. I have personally done it both ways, and while I prefer the ghee and enema option as I feel that I benefit from losing my appetite and resting, I have still had great results without them.

Elimination

Shutting down the digestion system means that you may cease to eliminate every day. If you become uncomfortable, you may take a few teaspoons of sesame oil or castor oil or drink senna tea. This will allow for morning elimination.

A Note of Caution

We perform the enemas at night so that the oil has a chance to soak into your system. You might be surprised that you receive the enema, go to bed, and get up in the morning having absorbed all of the oil. That's the perfect situation! Some people find that they are stimulated to immediately go to the bathroom, or they go to the bathroom in the morning and find that some oil does come out.

One of my participants did her enema in the morning and thought it absorbed, so she went to work. She sneezed violently at work and was surprised to find that it came out! Please keep a change of clothing in the car just in case.

Week 4 Overview

Rest and Relax

Week 4 is the week of YOU! This week you will be experiencing daily yoga, meditation twice daily of twenty minutes each, solitude, silence, and an easy-to-digest healing diet.

Follow the Cleansing Diet all week. Only eat when you are hungry. You may find that you are skipping meals or eating very little at mealtime. This is perfect. At some point during this week your digestive fire will ignite and you will be hungry! That is the signal that your Cleanse is coming to completion.

Do try to eat the Cleansing Diet for the full seven days. I've noticed over the years that The Winds usually eat it for three or four days and are done. The Fires will eat it for seven days because they are told to and The Earths or those needing to lose weight or shift disease will eat it up to fourteen days. I've had many Cleansers lose in excess of twenty pounds by extending the Cleanse.

This week we discuss coming off the Cleanse. Read this section carefully. The most important part of coming off the Cleanse is to mentally prepare the night before. Do not come off your Cleanse in the middle of the day. You will make bad choices, including indulging in less-favorable foods, and suffer. When you decide you are done, go to bed that night and set the intention that you are coming off of your Cleanse. Begin the process the following morning.

Revisit any of the spiritual exercises that you have not spent adequate time on. Every part of this program works together. We are building a foundation for physical, emotional, and spiritual health. It begins by cleaning out the body and calming the mind and ends with a powerful connection to Spirit. You have to have all the pieces of the puzzle in place to be happy.

If you have done your spiritual exercises, you are in the perfect place to spend some time this week writing your story. I want you to take your quiet time to journal your life. Use "The Good, the Bad, and the Ugly" as a foundation for your story up to this point. Use your intentions and desires to build your future. Think big. Think mythical. Let your story be the life of your dreams.

Many people struggle to think mythically. If that is the case for you, find some heroes from movies, books and real life to admire. Look to how they have accomplished their goals and write your story with their journey in mind. This will really inspire you. My heroes include Mother Teresa, Jesus, Buddha, Einstein, Deepak Chopra, Mark Whitwell, my children, my yogis, and more. I take pieces of their personality and life and fill in the gaps of my own story.

The most important thing to focus on this week is resting and relaxing. All of your activities should be nurturing and healing. Consider having a professional Ayurvedic massage this week. Choose gentle and nourishing yoga classes. Focus on yourself.

Have a great week.

Week 4 at a Glance
For Your Body

- Only eat when you are hungry. You do not need to eat three meals each day or eat at the same time each day.
- Follow the Week 4 eating plan. Legumes, white or brown rice, and vegetables.
- This is a vegan week. No meat, no dairy, and go light on fruit.
- Drink ginger tea. Sip this throughout your day. Use fresh ginger.
- Continue herbal therapy.
- Continue daily self-massage and receive professional massage.
- Continue daily movement that is gentle and nourishing all week.

For Your Mind

- Daily meditation of twenty minutes two times a day for a total of forty minutes. Continue to use the mantra, "so hum." Continue to begin your meditation with your questions: "Who am I?" "What do I want?" "How can I help and how can I serve?"
- Follow the daily routine. If you need to nap, do so this week.

For Your Spirit

- Daily silence. Drive in silence, cook in silence, and get ready for work in the morning in silence. Experience one hour of no talking each day.
- Spend some time in nature daily. This can be your thirty-minute walk.
- Write your story. Be mythical.
- Work every single day on your intentions and desires
- Journal every day.

It All Works Together
You Must Do Your Work on All Levels

Only you know the reason that you chose to participate in this program. Perhaps you are suffering weight gain, disease, fatigue, irritability, lack of joy or a calling from spirit to connect that has left you spinning. Regardless of why you came, the solution is the same for all. Do your work. Not one part of this program works independent of the other.

I know many people who meditate and pray daily but have poor health due to a lack of movement and poor food choices. They are not happy.

I know many people who are in great physical shape with active bodies, but they do not meditate, pray, or have a relationship with Spirit. They are not happy.

I know many people who meditate, pray, and have great bodies, but they will not face the dragons of their past. They are not happy.

My wish is that after the Cleanse ends, you will continue on your own. Do all the work of this program happily, knowing your journey never ends. You will continue to unfold just like a flower as you go deeper and deeper into your psyche. You are building a ladder that will take you to enlightenment or happiness.

During the Cleanse, you have established a foundation for your physical body through nutrition and movement. This will return you to balance and keep you healthy. You have cleaned out your covering made of food and boosted the metabolism of your tissues. Once your body feels good, you will no longer have to worry about it and you will be one step closer to happiness.

During the Cleanse, you have established a foundation for stress-reduction and spiritual connection through silence, mindfulness, and meditation. You have de-cluttered your brain of negative and useless thinking. You have learned a powerful tool to relax and to connect to spirit. You have cleaned out your emotional body. All energy channels of your body are now open. Now that you are aware of your thoughts and your ability to control them, you no longer have to let anxiety, worry, fear, anger, resentment, or betrayal rule your life. You are one step closer to happiness.

During the Cleanse you slayed the dragons of the past through the exercise called "The Good, the Bad, and the Ugly." This has allowed you to accept your current situation, to find the blessings in the not-so-wonderful things that sometimes happen, and to foster forgiveness and compassion for yourself and others involved in these pivotal moments. Now you can let the past go and with it let go of false ideas and beliefs that are holding you back. You are one step closer to happiness.

During the Cleanse you participated in an exercise called "Ego, I'd Like You to Meet Soul." This exercise made you aware of your sattvic (pure) qualities. It allowed you to cultivate them through daily meditation and daily focus. Your challenging qualities were identified as the ego qualities that are no longer serving you. You have learned to love your ego just as you do your soul, but you are not going to react from ego anymore. You will sit with emotions as they come up, honor them, and respond from a soul level. This releases you from creating drama, stress, and more karma in your life. You are one step closer to happiness.

During the Cleanse you participated in an exercise that connected you to your intentions and desires. This exercise allowed you to define your intentions and desires for this life. It allowed you permission to want what you want and accept that you deserve it. You now realize that your material and emotional needs are part of your journey. You deserve what you desire and you can create what you desire simply by putting focused attention and energy on what you want. You are one step closer to happiness.

During the Cleanse you participated in an exercise called "Karma Busting." This exercise allowed you to quickly identify what is your biggest obstacle to happiness, what will happen in your life if you don't change it, and what will happen in your life if you do. You have committed to self-study, deeply looking into your psyche to find and destroy that hidden choice-maker that is no longer serving you. You are one step closer to eliminating that obstacle that is serving you the least and holding you back from realizing happiness. You are one step closer to happiness.

During the Cleanse you participated in an exercise called "Write Your Story." This exercise allowed you to incorporate all of the above into a mythical story of your life. It allowed you the opportunity to dream big and connect with your life's purpose. You now realize that you are meant to live a mythical life. You are one step closer to happiness.

Embrace your new life. Be happy.

Coming Off Your Cleanse

Eat Consciously

Intend to take the Cleanse for the full seven days. I have noticed that The Winds (mind and body) tend to be done after four or five days. The Fires will take it the full seven days. The Earths will often take it well beyond the seven days.

If you are trying to shift weight or disease, do take it beyond the seven days if you can. I've had Cleansers take it up to fourteen days with incredible results of weight loss beyond twenty pounds. You will really benefit from this healing Cleansing diet.

At some point, you will feel done. When you find that your digestion has really turned back on and you are very hungry, you are done. Don't come off your Cleanse in the middle of the day or in the evening. Instead, tell yourself before you go to bed that you are ready to come off your Cleanse in the morning. This is very important. Most people who come off their Cleanse in an unplanned manner or at lunch or dinner will overindulge and feel really bad.

Your body is very sensitive at this point. If you consume meat, sugar, alcohol, greasy food, or caffeine, you will really feel it and possibly be sick.

For the first five days of returning to your life, you will drink the Yogi Breakfast for breakfast. We do this for two reasons. First, it is easily digestible, and second, it will keep you off your morning coffee for a little bit longer.

Slowly begin to add foods back into your diet, avoiding snacking. The foods you add back will be for your body type. All the foods you add back will incorporate your new lifestyle of whole, organic, local, and fresh. If you give up anything permanently, I hope it is red meat and milk. I also hope you use caution around sugar, caffeine, and alcohol.

Eat consciously. Feel your body accepting food. You will be amazed at the zip you get from that first cup of coffee, the buzz from the first glass of wine, the spike and crash from that first piece of cake, and the belly ache from that first fast food meal. You are in such a great space to accept the foods that are right for your body type, so don't mess it up by going back to less favorable habits.

Let your appetite return naturally; you may find yourself eating less for many days. At some point, you may find yourself incredibly hungry. That's a great sign! Your agni is high.

Live Consciously

Return to the world with care. Just as your body is sensitive, so is your mind. Continue to keep noise and chaos to a minimum. If you are planning outings and events, choose those that are more intimate and that involve people and situations you really care about.

I look at each of my 365 nights a year as special. When making plans, I always pause and ask if that is really how I want to spend 1 of the 365 nights of my year, knowing that I'll never get that night back. That little pause keeps me from doing a lot of things that I know I wouldn't really enjoy.

If you stop your meditation practice, you will notice that your life will begin to spin out of control. Don't worry. Simply sit back down on your chair and start over. If you quit entirely, you will notice a dramatic decline in your well-being.

I hope you continue to work on your intentions. Pull your journal out once a week and refresh. Notice what you have manifested and add to your list. This is a fun practice for life.

We'll talk more about how to live to balance your mind later.

Enjoy!

OM Work, Week 4: Write Your Creation Story

In every great spiritual tradition, there is a creation story. You have a creation story as well. Each story starts with an idea of Spirit and ends with a human on a journey. You are a thought of God. You are divinity expressing through.

The creation story of Ayurveda is that there is something that exists that we could never begin to understand. This is called Brahman. It is total nothingness of a nature that the human mind can't conceive. It is before creation. Within this nothingness lives an energy called Parusha. I like to think of Parusha as a wise older brother sitting in a meditative stance. Parusha is the ultimate observer. Parusha simply looks on and observes.

Parusha observes his younger sister, Prakruti. Prakruti is much like the Fool from the Tarot deck. One foot rests in the unmanifest and one foot rests in the manifest. Prakruti is a showoff. She wants to entertain Parusha, so when she becomes aware that she is being observed, she steps off the edge of the cliff and manifestation or creation begins.

At this point, consciousness becomes matter and the creative intelligence or the brain of creation forms, and this is called Mahad. Mahad contains all of intelligence and is aware of itself. Mahad organizes and creates structure. The millisecond Mahad becomes buddhi or aware of itself through intellect it becomes Ahamkara, or the ego. Ahamkara has a sense of "I am." It is separate. It observes what is around it and understands that it is separate of its observations. This is the point of your human birth. You come to this world Mahad knowing yourself as complete. Intellect takes over and you bring the world to focus through senses and perceive that you are separate. As you grow, your perception of your separateness increases as the layers of maya (illusion) engulf you. Ignorance or non-remembering your divinity begins. Ignorance is at the root of all suffering.

Energizing all of this is prana. Prana is the flow of cosmic energy. Think of it as blood flow on a subtle level, the heartbeat of the universe. The vibrations that the universe make as it spins through space pulse prana in the same way blood pulses through veins. The rotation of the planets changes the pulse, subtly affecting you individually.

These pulsations of prana break creation into the gunas of sattva, rajas, and tamas. The gunas allow us to experience this reality as tangible through the expression of the elements: Space, Air, Water, Fire, and Earth. We experience these with our senses, and they create the illusion (maya) of our existence.

The point of this esoteric discourse is that the minute you were born, you knew that you were part of something bigger. The more time you spent in the world, the more time you became deluded by illusion and decided you were separate. As a child, you were so close to oneness that you knew yourself as perfect. You operated from a heart-centered place and made spontaneous right choices. You were yoga, or joined in your higher heart. That's who you are.

You are remembering. Depending on your experiences from childhood and life, you may be more or less off center of your higher heart. Every situation in your life has the potential to pull you off center. Yoga is the process of bringing you back to center. My intention for The Elemental Cleanse is to empower you to bring yourself back to center.

At this point in the Cleanse, Week 4, you are in a very powerful place to pull the pieces of your life together and dream big for your future. You have a clearer understanding of the past, you understand your ego and soul qualities, you have a vision for the things in your life that you desire to manifest, and you are beginning to understand that your life has purposes and meaning.

Now you simply need to remember who you are.

Gather all of your Om Work from the other weeks. During this final week of quiet reflection and solitude, write your creation story. Begin with your childhood, remembering your perfection. Gaze into the eyes of the child in that picture that is sitting on your altar and remember what it was like to be so small and perfect.

Add to your story the situations in your life that began to pull you off center. This information is found in "The Good, the Bad, and the Ugly." Release the negativity of the past and intend to not allow these situations to affect your future.

Write about yourself. You are aware of the sattvic qualities of your soul and ego that you want to express. Create a profile of this beautiful person with whom you are connecting.

Finish the story of your life by writing about all the things and situations you intend for your future. Connect the dots between your intentions and your life's purpose. Be mythical. If you struggle with this, look to our cultural archetypes for inspiration and model your life after theirs.

Make this process fun. I've had participants do this in many forms. Some have written a page and some a book. Some have even used a creative outlet like painting to express their story. You will find this process to be empowering and a beautiful work to come back to if and when you find you are off your path.

Living in Balance

ongratulations, you did it! I'm so happy for you, and I hope that you feel wonderful. This next section is about how to maintain your state of balance by embracing the nutrition and lifestyle that is right for your body and mind.

First, though, I'd like you to retake your balance quiz to make sure that you have come back to balance. Scores in any area of eleven or less indicate balance. If you have not returned to balance, scan the self-assessment quiz included in this section to quickly determine what parts of the Cleanse need more attention. Some people find that their focus went one way or another and they neglected certain aspects such as meditation, yoga, or the spiritual exercises, and they simply need to incorporate more of these to come back to balance.

If you were shifting an Earth imbalance such as weight gain, know that it is simply going to take more time. You may stay with the Cleansing Diet for one more week, but then it is time to begin to eat for your body type or to follow The Earth eating plan to continue to shift weight. Healthy weight loss that is sustainable is losing one to two pounds per week.

This section includes a discussion of the tastes of Ayurveda and how they affect your body type. You will find that eating for your body type is not that difficult. The most important thing to know is that there are no bad foods. However, much of what we eat is so over-processed it no longer retains nutritional value and can hardly be called food. If you simply understand the following, you have come a long way:

- Food is to be organic, local, and whole.
- Food is primarily beans, vegetables, whole grains, fruits, nuts, seeds, and oils.
- Food is consumed in a settled environment at regular times and eaten consciously.
- You must grocery shop and cook to maintain balance.
- A meal consists of about two cups of food.
- In your stomach lives your digestive fire (agni). Keep that fire stoked to maximize digestion and metabolism.
- In your mind lives your digestive fire (agni). Put positive thoughts, good choices, healthy relationships, and meaningful jobs in your mind to keep digestion at its maximum.
- Your health—physical, mental, and spiritual—is critical to achieving happiness.

153

Use the Self-Assessment Quiz as a way to monitor your daily balance. Take the balance quizzes every twenty-one days to make sure that you are on track. Remember that 90 percent of disease can be easily treated with nutrition and routine. Most of these diseases are due to an imbalance of The Wind (Vata) in your body or mind. When you feel this imbalance settling in, take immediate action to adjust your lifestyle and you will prevent deeper diseases.

I urge you to Cleanse your body on an annual basis. I have many students who come back year after year. I personally have been living this lifestyle for ten years and am still unfolding layers of thought and habit. Your work never ends.

On a monthly basis, you can experience a mini two or three day Cleanse. It's simple! If you are female, time it with the end of your menstrual cycle. If you are male or if you no longer menstruate, time it with the full moon.

Mini Cleanse

- Do not give up any of your habits. This will stress your system with withdrawal. Have consciousness around your habits and if you can easily skip something, do so.
- Take neem and triphala. Do not worry about guggulu. It needs more than three days to be effective.
- Live in silence. Turn off the media, the TV, and the radio and keep talking to a minimum.
- Revisit the eating routine and nature's routine. Use the self-assessment quiz to guide you.
- Critical for a mini-cleanse is eating three meals each day around the same time and going to bed by 10:00 p.m.
- Eat the Cleansing Diet.
- Drink ginger tea.
- Go to yoga every day.
- Meditate every day for no fewer than twenty minutes.

The Balance Quiz

Do you balance? Answer how you have been feeling the past twenty-one days using the following scale.

1. NOT AT ALL
2. LITTLE BIT
3. SOMEWHAT
4. MODERATELY
5. VERY MUCH

— I've been having trouble concentrating. I am forgetful.

— I have been talking a lot and having trouble listening.

— I have been having trouble sleeping. I can't go to sleep, or I wake up and can't fall back to sleep.

— I have been very worried lately.

— I can't seem to stick to a routine. I am impulsive.

— **The Wind in Your Mind (total)**

— I have no routine. I eat, sleep, and perform activities at inconsistent times each day.

— I am suffering from gas and bloating.

— I have constipation. My elimination is hard and dry.

— I have been suffering from a lot of situations; back pain, headaches.

— My skin, nail, and hair feel dry.

— **The Wind in Your Body (total)**

— I have been very impatient lately.

— I am critical and judgmental.

— I have been very opinionated and forceful in sharing my opinion.

— I feel like others simply aren't doing a good job and I need to be in charge.

— I have been losing my temper.

— **The Fire in Your Mind (total)**

— My skin is suffering from outbreaks, rashes, and inflammation.

— I have heartburn or indigestion.

— I have hot flashes.

— I have loose elimination.

— My breath seems bad. My body odor is sour.

— **The Fire in Your Body (total)**

— I have been quiet and withdrawn. I do not want to deal with conflict.

— My thoughts are dull. I don't want to try new things.

— I feel jealous, possessive, and needy.

— I want to make changes, but I just can't.

— I feel depressed.

— **The Earth in Your Mind (total)**

— I've been gaining weight and holding it.

— I feel sluggish in the morning and want to sleep in.

— I have sinus congestion, nasal allergies or asthma.

— I am retaining fluids.

— **The Earth in Your Body (total)**

If your scores are in the 5–9 range in any individual category, you are in balance. If your scores are 10–15, you have a moderate imbalance. If your scores are above 15, you are out of balance. If you have anything above 10, you should continue to Cleanse.

You have completed your balance quiz and hopefully you have returned to a state of balance. If you have returned to a state of balance, congratulations. You may begin to follow your dosha's plan for living in balance.

If you have not returned to balance, please review the Self-Assessment Quiz on the following pages. Notice the parts of the Cleanse that you did not adhere to or focus on. You may see that there are one or two practices that require more focus in the next week or two.

If you are not in balance, you may extend the Cleanse. Continue to eat the Cleansing Diet for one more week and then take the quiz again. This, coupled with yoga, meditation, and silence should bring you back to balance. If you are shifting weight or disease, it is beneficial to extend the Cleanse for one more week. After that week, eat for your imbalance, or if you are back in balance, eat for your dosha.

The Self-Assessment Quiz on the following pages can be used as a guide for life. If you notice that you are mentally or physically going out of balance, refer back to this quiz to see if any of your habits have returned or if any of your practices are neglected.

Self-Assessment Quiz

Use this list to stay on track for life. Turn it into a twenty-one-day worksheet for your refrigerator.

I was in bed by 10:00 p.m.

I was up by 5:00–7:00 a.m.

I drank a glass of water upon rising.

I ate breakfast within one hour of rising.

I self-massaged.

I took my herbal therapy.

I drank ginger tea.

Lunch was my largest meal.

Each meal was no more than two cups.

I chose healthy snacks.

I avoided meat.

I avoided caffeine.

I walked for thirty minutes.

I meditated for twenty minutes.

I enjoyed nature.

My food satisfied me today.

I feel good about the food choices I made today.

I did not eat for reasons other than hunger.

My food and other choices contributed to my higher good.

My food and other choices contributed to the realization of my dharma.

I prayed today.

I expressed gratitude.

I journaled.

I used affirmation today instead of unnecessary thought.

I focused mindfully on breath.

I practiced loving kindness and compassion.

I was helpful.

I spoke kindly to myself.

The Tastes of Ayurveda

Building Blocks for Nutrition

Let's begin the process of learning how to eat for our body types. Ayurveda categorizes the sensation, satisfaction, and emotional component of eating into six tastes. Depending on your predominant nature, you will favor three of the six tastes and minimize the other three. Note that I stress *minimize;* I did not say *eliminate*. All six tastes must be present in your diet to promote a feeling of satisfaction. The tastes are sweet, sour, salty, pungent, bitter, and astringent.

The Sweet Taste: Cools, Creates Heaviness, and Is Oily

The sweet taste is made from the elements Earth and Water. That means that if you are made from a predominance of these elements, you have a lot of sweet in you. This is The Earth (Kapha) dosha. Common sources are grains, dairy, breads, pasta, starchy vegetables, fruits, nuts, oils, sugar, honey, and meat.

The sweet taste builds tissue and is the most nutritive. It relieves both hunger and thirst. Taken in excess, the sweet taste leads to obesity, heart disease, diabetes, laziness, congestion, poor circulation, inflammation, indigestion, gas and bloating, allergies, and respiratory illness, including too much mucus. Mentally, excess sweet taste leads to lethargy, dullness, and greed.

If you are The Wind, this taste is very grounding and nourishing. You can eat an abundance of this taste. In fact, the taste of sweet will be your primary source of calories. The Wind is a person who has a difficult time gaining weight. The abundance of calories found in this taste do not affect a balanced Wind. The Wind can eat dairy and meat. I caution you to only consume three to five servings of meat each week that is organic, local, and fresh. Avoid red meat all together.

If you are The Fire, this taste is very cooling to you. You can eat an abundance of this taste. While you are going to find your primary source of calories from beans and vegetables, you will consume a fair quantity of sweet. Fires make the best vegetarians, but do benefit from dairy. In fact, Fires should treat themselves to an ice cream cone once in a while.

If you are The Earth, this heavy and dense taste is going to create imbalance. Minimize this taste. In fact, Earths should avoid dairy and meat altogether. When consuming, know that you should spice your sweet taste with pungent spices. Adding cinnamon or nutmeg to dairy is a way to enhance digestion. Think of your meat as a condiment. Season and spice and work into your food as an ingredient, just as they do at a Thai restaurant.

The Salty Taste: Creates Heaviness and Heat and Is Oily

The salty taste is made of the elements Water and Fire. That means if you are made of a predominance of these elements, you have a lot of the salty taste. The Fire (Pitta) and The Earth (Kapha) both contain a lot of salt. Common sources are salt, seafood, sauces, and meat.

The salty taste stimulates digestion. It cleanses the body by softening and loosening the tissues. It makes other foods taste better. Taken in excess, the salty taste leads to bloating, inflammation, skin disorders, bleeding, joint disease, premature wrinkling, baldness, and impotence. Mentally, excess salt leads to overindulgence.

If you are The Wind, this taste is balancing. In fact, many Winds crave salty and crunchy snacks. There is no recommended allowance for salt intake. Buy an organic iodized salt and feel free to cook with this spice.

If you are The Fire, this taste should be minimized. The excess heat in salt leads to upset belly, indigestion, heartburn, and anger. Everyone needs the iodine added to salt, but use it sparingly when you cook and do not salt your food.

If you are The Earth, this taste should be minimized. Excess salt leads to bloating in this body type. Everyone needs the iodine added to salt, but use it sparingly when you cook and do not salt your food.

The Sour Taste: Creates Heat and Heaviness and Is Oily

The Sour Taste is composed of the elements Earth and Fire. That means if you are made of a predominance of these elements, you have a lot of the sour taste in you. The Earth (Kapha) and The Fire (Pitta) have a lot of this taste in them. Sources are citrus fruits, sour fruits, tomatoes, yogurt, cheese, pickles, vinegar, and alcohol.

The sour taste is acidic. It stimulates digestion and is suggested for those trying to improve digestion. It refreshes the senses. In excess, the sour taste leads to burning sensations, aging, and itching. Mentally, it causes jealousy and a lack of caring for the things that you have in your life.

If you are The Wind, this is a balancing taste. In fact, this taste helps The Wind to maintain digestive fire. Feel free to eat yogurt for breakfast, and add lemon to your waters and teas.

If you are The Fire, the heat in this taste can lead to acid indigestion, heartburn, or a sour belly. Many Fires have no problem with this taste, however, so please consume the taste of sour consciously and notice how it affects you. I find that the sour taste is difficult to overindulge in and usually treat it as an ingredient, thereby minimizing its impact on The Fire digestion.

If you are The Earth, the moisture in this taste can lead to bloating and sluggish digestion. Minimize this taste.

The Pungent or Spicy Taste: Creates Heat, Lightness, and Dryness

The spicy taste is made from the elements Fire and Air. That means if you are made from a predominance of these elements, you have a lot of spice in you. The Fire (Pitta) and The Wind (Vata) are made from this taste.

Common sources are peppers, ginger, salsa, mustard, basil, and thyme.

The pungent taste stimulates digestion, clears congestion, and detoxifies the body. It has the ability to flush mucus and fat from the body. In excess, the pungent taste leads to thirst, emaciation, burning, pain, dryness, fever, and dizziness. Mentally, it leads to impatience and anger.

If you are The Wind, minimize this taste. The Wind has delicate digestion and can greatly benefit from a little pungent spice to stoke the digestive fire, but in excess this can lead to an upset belly. Eat the taste of pungent consciously until you figure out what spice level is right for you.

If you are The Fire, minimize this taste. The Fire already has heated digestion. Even just a little bit of the pungent taste can give The Fire heartburn, indigestion, and even diarrhea. Eat this taste consciously until you figure out what spice level is right for you.

If you are The Earth, maximize this taste. The Earth is going to thrive on pungent spices. Because The Earth is choosing a diet of mostly grains, beans, and vegetables, the pungent spices are going to add a lot of complexity and satisfaction to meals. The pungent spices are also going to stoke a sluggish digestive fire and facilitate elimination. Be bold and get creative in the kitchen with spice.

The Bitter Taste: Cools and Creates Lightness and Dryness

The bitter taste is composed of the elements Air and Space. If you have a predominance of these elements, you contain a lot of this taste. The Wind (Vata) is made from this taste. Common sources are green and yellow vegetables and green leafy vegetables.

The bitter taste acts as an anti-inflammatory and detoxifies the body. It dries secretions like mucus. It is wonderful for skin disorders. The herb neem that you are taking as part of your Cleanse is the bitter taste. In excess, the bitter taste leads to headache, constipation, aches and pains, insomnia and sleeplessness, dryness, emaciation, tremors, and stiffness. Mentally it can lead to dissatisfaction.

If you are The Wind, minimize this taste. You are already very uplifted and need to focus on grounding your energy. You do need to consume vegetables, but always cook them first in a little oil or ghee to make them dense. A wonderful trick is to add a little goat cheese or feta to your vegetables. Always eat your salads at room temperature and add oil, nuts, and seeds for balance.

If you are The Fire, maximize this taste. In fact, Fires make wonderful vegetarians and thrive on vegetables. Fires have strong enough digestion that they may eat their vegetables cold and raw.

If you are The Earth, maximize this taste. Do cook your vegetables prior to consumption. Focus on dry cooking methods like roasting or steaming instead of sautéing in oil or ghee. Spice up your vegetables with pungent spices to make them more interesting.

The Astringent Taste: Cools and Creates Lightness and Dryness

The astringent taste is more like a sensation. Think about how your mouth feels after you've eaten an unripe banana or spinach.

The astringent taste is made from the elements Air and Earth (tiny little bit). If you have a predominance of these elements in your body, you are made of this taste. The Wind (Vata) has an abundance of this taste. The Earth (Kapha), however, does not, even though this taste is made from a tiny bit of Earth.

Common sources are beans, legumes, lentils, pomegranates, cranberries, tea, and dark greens.

The astringent taste promotes healing. It purifies. It dries all secretions. Overindulgence in the astringent taste can lead to headache, constipation, aches and pains, insomnia and sleeplessness, dryness, emaciation, tremors, stiffness, and thirst. Mentally, it leads to anxiety and fear.

If you are The Wind, minimize this taste. It is an uplifting taste, and The Wind needs to focus on foods to ground and nourish the body. Because The Wind has delicate digestion, beans can be very hard to digest and can lead to gas, bloating, and constipation. Choose only those beans that can be cooked in less than thirty minutes without soaking. This includes lentils, dal, dahl, and split peas.

If you are The Fire, maximize this taste. The Fire is a vegetarian and thrives on all kinds of beans. Your strong digestion can handle all beans, including those with thick skins like kidney beans.

If you are The Earth, maximize this taste. Add pungent spices to facilitate strong digestion. Depending upon the individual, Earths may find that they prefer beans that have thinner skins and cook more quickly. Test out all beans and learn to love them.

The following table shows the best tastes for balancing each element.

	The Wind	**The Fire**	**The Earth**
Best Taste	Salty	Bitter	Spicy
2nd Best	Sour	Sweet	Bitter
3rd Best	Sweet	Astringent	Astringent

This chart is helpful for you to cook your food and to choose proportionate eating. You now know that if you are The Wind, you should use salt and citrus when cooking to prepare your body to digest. You will choose grains and pastas. Go easy on the bread. Many Winds experience gas and bloating from bread due to its yeasty content.

If you are The Fire, you are going to favor the taste of leafy greens and have a bigger serving of these than of grains and pastas. You also know that beans are one of your best dishes.

The Earth is going to really spice up its food, favoring vegetables and beans. The sweet taste is the worse taste for the Earth. Go very lightly on the breads and pastas. Meat and dairy are to be avoided.

Your Senses

We enjoy all six tastes and feel satisfaction only when we have not overindulged our five senses of taste, touch, sight, hearing, and smell. For this reason, the natural routine and eating routine are very important. If your senses are overstimulated, you will not be able to enjoy your food and you will overindulge. Enjoy your food. Enjoy your life. Not being able to discern taste is the first sign of imbalance.

Your Emotions

I know it seems crazy, but food does affect your emotions. For example, too much of the sweet taste will create dullness and lethargy. Think about the last weekend or vacation you took during which you overindulged in sweet. It left you feeling a little dull, maybe even depressed. Pay attention to the foods you are choosing and why. Pay attention to the emotional eating that you engage in. The sweet taste has a lot of love and comfort in it. We indulge in it to feel love.

If you have situations around cravings and food, start to incorporate your experience into a journal and see if you have a habit or emotional pattern.

An Overview of Eating for Your Dosha

You have learned a lot about eating for your dosha over the past twenty-eight days. If you were consuming a relatively healthy American diet with a little bit of meat and dairy, you were already eating for The Wind (Vata). As you moved toward the elimination of meat but were still eating some dairy, you were eating for The Fire (Pitta). As you began to add pungent spices and totally eliminate meat and dairy, you were eating for The Earth (Kapha).

Take a moment to think over the past twenty-eight days. What part of the Cleanse resonated with you the most? What did you crave or miss? Chances are, if you were craving salty snacks, you are a Vata. If you were craving iced beverages, you are a Pitta, and if you were craving sweets, you are a Kapha.

The following discussion on living for each body and mind type is broken up according to dosha. Read each section. The key to living in balance in not just to eat and live for your type, but also to understand that you have the other doshas in you and sometimes they go out of balance. For example, if you find yourself not sleeping, having a hard time concentrating, and suffering from aches and pains, chances are your Vata is out of balance and you need to switch to that lifestyle for a few days until you come back to balance. If you are suffering from irritability, heartburn, indigestion, or loose elimination, chances are your Pitta is out of balance and you need to switch to that lifestyle for a few days until you come back to balance. If you find yourself with respiratory conditions and are lethargic, depressed, or sluggish in the bathroom, chances are your Kapha is out of balance and you need to switch to that lifestyle for more than a few days.

It's really powerful to understand that Vata is the first dosha to go out of balance and is easily pulled back to balance with routine and nutrition. If you could catch every imbalance at the initial onset, you would never go very far out of balance.

The Wind Living in Balance

Ground the Force of The Wind

If you are The Wind, the key to living in balance is routine. I know you resist routine and dislike it. However, it is the absolute best thing you can do for yourself.

The following are common situations you may be prone to because you are The Wind. If you are The Fire or The Earth, you may also experience these situations and should follow The Wind Living in Balance plan until the situation passes.

- Insomnia or sleeplessness
- Tremors or shakiness
- Constipation
- IBS
- Most headaches
- Back pain
- Stress from traveling
- Anytime you have surgery
- Anxiety and worry

The following is the ideal routine for The Wind (or for a Wind situation). Stick to it as much as possible. Definitely stick to it when you feel the Wind going out of balance in your mind or body. How will you know when you are going out of balance? You will experience racing thoughts, anxiety, worry, nervousness, and sleeplessness. You may experience headaches, backaches, constipation, nervous tremors, or aches and pains. If you immediately adjust your routine, you can eliminate these symptoms and prevent deeper disease.

Routine for The Wind (Vata Dosha) in Mind

Minimize noise and chaos in your environment. Please participate in a media blackout. This includes TV, radio, and much of our current communication mechanisms including e-mail, Facebook, texting, and excessive cell phone usage or monitoring.

Avoid unnecessary conversation and events. Stay home. Be alone and rest. If an event is chaotic and loud or includes meeting a lot of new people, don't go. Say no. Avoid shopping malls and crowds.

Instead, choose quiet places if you want to get out: libraries and bookstores, art museums, tea houses, lunch/dinner with close friends.

Participate in gentle or restorative yoga class each week. You also love walking, leisurely biking, hiking, and martial arts practices such as Tai Chi and Qi Gong. All are gentle and nourishing.

Stay warm, avoiding drafts and wind. Cover your face with a scarf when you go outside. Wear mittens. Warm your car up before you get in. Favor colors that are earthy and rich: browns, oranges, yellows, and greens.

Darken your environment. Keep lights low. Light candles. Burn candles, incense, and essential oils that are warm and grounding: ylang ylang, sandalwood, frankincense, neroli, musk, lavender, and vanilla. Listen to grounding and soothing music. Classical music is perfect for Vata! Treat yourself to hot baths, steam rooms, saunas and a massage.

Get dirty. Make a mess in your kitchen, dig in the earth, and spend time nourishing your family.

Honoring that you like to flit from thing to thing and creatively thrive in a bit of chaos is okay. You can still step back and look at your week and schedule routine into it. At the beginning of each week, sit down with your schedule and plan your week. This step alone can save you from some of the chaos of living.

What to Eat

Eating to balance The Wind means that you are going to favor heavy, dense, and grounding foods. Favor the sweet, sour, and salty tastes.

That's great news for you, because those are the tastes of the American diet that we are all accustomed to. You are able to eat more meat, dairy, pasta, whole grains, citrus fruits, fermented foods, and salt.

Don't get up and do a little dance just yet though. When I say you can eat meat, I mean only three to five servings a week. A serving is the size of the palm of your hand. Please give up red meat, including beef and pork, entirely. Favor poultry and fish that is sustainably farmed, organic, and free range…that had a nice life. The pasta and grains you are choosing should be organic and whole. We still don't want the color white in our diet.

Critical Success Factors to Healthy Wind Digestion

- Eat three meals each day around the same time each day.
- Some Winds do better eating four meals each day, allowing at least two hours between each meal. Try it and see if it agrees with you. Eat small amounts.
- Eat within one hour of rising.
- Lunch is your biggest meal and includes meat if you are choosing to eat meat.
- Foods are warm, moist, and cooked. You thrive on casseroles, stews, and food that has been mixed together and cooked.
- No eating two to three hours before bedtime.
- If you do snack, you should allow two hours between snacks and meals.
- You really benefit from a short walk after your meal.
- You benefit greatly by placing a glass of water by your bedside each evening and drinking it down first thing in the morning.
- Favor foods in the following order:
  1. Whole grains
  2. Cooked vegetables
  3. Beans that cook in less than thirty minutes without soaking
  4. Cooked fruits
  5. Nuts, seeds, honey, and oils
  6. Spice to taste; salt is okay

- You may consume dairy in the form of milk, yogurt, and soft cheeses like feta and goat. Do notice if yogurt and milk agree with you. Many Vatas are sensitive to these dairy products.

The following lists include items that your body type typically digests very well or not so well. Please eat consciously and simply notice if the foods aggravate you or appeal to you. Just because a food item appears on this list under avoid does not mean that you will be affected negatively by it. You have all the forces in your body; some other force may be helping you specifically to digest and enjoy items on the avoid side.

Fruits:

Favor (heavy and dense)

Mangos
Dates

Oranges
Bananas
Grapes
Grapefruit
Apricots
Avocados
Papaya
Peaches

Avoid (light and crisp)

Dried fruits
Cranberries
Pomegranates
Apples

Vegetables:
Favor

Sweet potatoes
Squash
Avocados
Carrots
Asparagus
Beets
Turnips, parsnips, radishes

Avoid
Raw vegetables
Onions
Broccoli
Cabbage
Cauliflower
Tomatoes

Beans and Legumes:

As a general rule, if it cooks in less than thirty minutes without soaking, The Wind digestion can handle it.
Favor
(split beans)

Mung beans
Lentils
Chickpeas
Tofu

Avoid
(Any bean with thick skin)
Black beans
Navy beans
Kidney beans

The Wind should always spice beans with turmeric, cumin, ginger, garlic, and a bit of oil or ghee to promote digestion.

Other:

Favor
Skinless almonds are the best
All nuts, best as butters
All oils
All dairy
All sweeteners
All spices except pungent
Diluted wine* with meal

Avoid
Hard cheese
White sweeteners
Pungent spices
Beer, hard liquor

*Know that the Wind is the most addictive of types. Use alcohol with caution and drink consciously.

The Fire Living in Balance

Pacify the Force of the Fire

If you are The Fire, the key to living in balance is to cool your body and mind. Find a way to release the heat that builds up.

The following are very common situations that you may be prone to because you are The Fire. If you are The Wind or The Earth, you may also experience these situations and should follow this plan until the situation passes:

- Heartburn or ulcers
- Diarrhea
- Bad breath or body odor
- Hemorrhoids
- Infection
- Rashes, acne, skin irritation
- Inflammation
- Canker sores
- Sore throat
- PMS
- Grumpiness, anger, impatience
- The need to control and be right

The following is the ideal routine for The Fire. Stick to it as much as possible. Definitely stick to it when you feel The Fire going out of balance in your mind or body. How will you know when you are going out of balance? You will experience hostility, rage, or irritation. You will believe that you are the only person who can do things right and will become critical of others. You may find yourself working excessively and becoming grumpy. You may experience pounding headaches, tension, stress, acid indigestion, hot flashes, heart palpitations, and high blood pressure.

Routine for The Fire (Pitta Dosha) in the Mind

Minimize noise and chaos in your environment. When you return from noise and chaos, give yourself ten minutes of quiet and solitude to cool down.

Participate daily in a vigorous exercise program that includes a ten-minute minimum rest to cool at the end. You must rest after vigorous activity. This is critical. You love vinyasa and ashtanga yoga practices that are physically challenging. Martial arts, hiking, biking, swimming, and running are all perfect. Swimming is one of the best things for you.

Include at least one gentle yoga practice a week in your exercise program. Yin and restorative are both good choices.

Spend time in nature. You thrive being outdoors.

Stay cool. Favor colors that are cooling and represent water; turquoise, mint green, soft pinks, yellows, and white. Darken your environment. Keep lights low. Burn incense and essential oils that are cooling and soothing: lily, honeysuckle, sandalwood, mint, lemongrass, gardenia, jasmine, lavender, and chamomile.

Avoid work-related stress. (This works for family stress too) Fires suffer enormously at work if they have bosses who do not empower them. Minimize and manage your stress at work by incorporating the following into your mind and environment:

- Arrive at work before rush hour and before coworkers. Use this time to quietly organize your day and make plans.
- Cool down your environment. Hang pictures of ocean scenes, buy a fish for your desk, and bring in plants. If you listen to music, choose sounds of the ocean or nature to quietly play in the background.
- If you are able to close your door at work, do so.
- Go for a walk outside at lunchtime. Get away from all coworkers.
- Relinquish your need to be right. Have three working plans in your mind and make sure you have flexibility around those plans. If someone makes a suggestion that fits into one of your plans, accept it.
- Drive home in silence and let your mind play out the events of the day. Simply observe them as if you are a witness. As emotions arise, simply notice them in a clinical and non-judgmental way. Be the observer.
- When you come home from work, greet your family with hugs and tell them you are going to take fifteen minutes to unwind. Go to a secluded spot and lie down in Shavasana for ten minutes. Rest, relax and let your day go so that you can enjoy your family.
- If your family greets you at the door with their troubles, just let them talk. Relinquish the need to provide advice and solutions. They just want to talk and get it out. Just listen and let it go.

You do love routine. Take time to schedule time for yourself daily. You require physical movement and solitude each day. Couple these needs with your love of the outdoors.

What to Eat

Eating to balance The Fire means that you are going to eat a larger proportion of the foods you are not made of. You are going to favor the bitter, astringent, and sweet tastes.

I want to stress that you are avoiding certain foods, but you don't have to entirely eliminate them. Eating all six tastes creates satisfaction. The Fire should, however, eliminate meat. This is not because you don't have the strong digestion necessary to digest meat, but because you are predisposed to heart disease, high blood pressure, and heart attack. Meat contains the most saturated fat and is known to contribute to heart disease and cancer.

Critical Success Factors to Healthy Fire Digestion

- Eat three meals each day around the same time each day. Leave four to six hours between meals.
- Eat within one hour of rising.
- Lunch is your biggest meal and includes meat if you are choosing to eat meat. Fires make good vegetarians. Meat is not your best choice.
- Foods are cool, dry, and cooked or raw. You can eat raw food.
- No eating two to three hours before bedtime.

- If you do snack, you should allow four hours between snacks and meals.
- You benefit from a short walk after your meal.
- Be careful not to overindulge. Your strong digestion appears to suffer little from it, but you will gain weight.
- Favor foods in the following order:
  1. All beans
  2. Vegetables, cooked or raw
  3. Whole grains
  4. Fruits
  5. Seeds

You may eat nuts, honey, and oil, but do note how they make you feel. Many Fires have a little bit of a belly upset after eating oily nuts, heating honey, and oily oil. Test it out and see how you feel.

Eat a more bland diet. Spicy spices may not agree with you. Salt is to be avoided, as it is too heating. If you currently consume these and are in balance and are not digestively disturbed, spice your food to taste.

You may consume dairy in the form of milk, yogurt, and soft cheeses like feta and goat.

The following lists include items that your body type typically digests very well or not so well. Please eat consciously and simply notice if the foods aggravate you or appeal to you. Just because a food item appears on this list under avoid does not mean that you will be affected negatively by it. You have all the forces in your body; some other force may be helping you specifically to digest and enjoy items on the avoid side.

Fruits:

Favor

All fruit except for citrus fruits

Avoid

(heavy and dense)
Citrus fruits

Vegetables:

Favor

All vegetables
Dandelion, gentian, golden seal, milk thistle, mugwort

Avoid

(none)

Beans and Legumes:

I'm not going to place any bean on the avoid side. Try out all kinds of beans, as beans are your staple. Notice if the thicker-skinned beans create gas and bloating. If you can't spice them and cook them to avoid gas and bloating, then put them on your avoid list.

More beans to try: adzuki, black, black-eyed peas, butter, cannellini, edamame, great northern, kidney, lima, navy, pinto, soy

Other:

Favor

Natural sweeteners
Spices that are not pungent
All dairy
All grains
Coconut oil
All nuts and seeds
Wine

Avoid

Honey (may be too heating)
Pungent spices and salt
Yogurt (if it upsets your belly)
Oil (use sparingly)
Beer and hard alcohol

The Fire loves amaranth, buckwheat, hempseed, soybeans, quinoa, and spirulina (take as supplement) because they are complete proteins.

The Earth Living in Balance

Uplift the force of The Earth. If you are The Earth, the key to living in balance is to move your body and mind, uplifting your energy.

The following are very common situations that you may be prone to because you are The Earth. If you are The Wind or The Fire, you may also experience these situations and should follow this plan until the situation passes:

- Respiratory illness
- Colds with deep cough
- Flu
- Asthma
- Bronchitis
- Swollen glands
- Excessive weight gain or obesity
- Diabetes
- Depression
- Cysts
- Arthritis
- Cancer
- Inflammatory conditions like fibromyalgia

The following is the ideal routine for The Earth. Stick to it as much as possible. Definitely stick to it when you feel The Earth going out of balance in your mind or body. How will you know when you are going out of balance? You will experience dullness, lethargy, pessimism, clinginess, and depression. You may experience sluggish bowels, weight gain, inflammation, allergies, sinuses, and bronchial passages. If you immediately adjust your routine, you can quickly eliminate these symptoms and prevent the long-term stay of these situations and, ultimately, deeper disease.

Go to bed by 11:00 p.m. and arise by 5:00 or 6:00 a.m. (Many Earths can even get up earlier!) Never sleep in. Avoid napping.

Turn up the stereo and try something invigorating…especially in the morning. Dance around or vigorously clean a room in your home. Participate daily in a vigorous exercise program that includes a ten-minute minimum rest at the end. You love vinyasa and ashtanga yoga practices that are physically challenging. Martial arts, hiking, biking, and running are all perfect. Dancing is one of the best hobbies you can experience.

Your walk in nature should be vigorous and stimulating. Walk during hours of light.

Make social plans with family and friends. Go out. Have fun. Try something new.

Declutter your home. If it seems overwhelming, simply get some boxes, put all clutter in the boxes, and move the boxes to the basement or closet to go through and make decisions about later.

Stay warm and dry. Seek out heat therapy that is dry, including saunas and sunshine.

Favor colors that are bright and uplifting; blues, greens, yellows, and reds.

Open the curtains and let the sunshine in! Light up your house. Burn candles, incense, and essential oils that are warming and stimulating: orange, peppermint, pine, jasmine, sage, and eucalyptus are all good choices.

Honoring that you love your routine is perfect. You can still step back and look at your week and schedule a little unpredictability into it. Carve out little blocks of time and allow them to fill up with lunch dates, new activities, and adventures. When people ask you to try something new with them, say yes. This step alone will save you from becoming lethargic.

What to Eat

Eating to balance The Earth means that you are going to favor light, spicy, and uplifting foods. You are going to favor the bitter, astringent, and pungent tastes of Ayurveda. The Earth thrives on a vegetarian diet.

I want to stress that you are avoiding certain foods, but you don't have to entirely eliminate them. Eating all six tastes creates satisfaction. The Earth should, however, avoid meat and dairy completely. Start by embracing a vegetarian lifestyle and don't worry too much about dairy content as an ingredient. It can be overwhelming to go from a regular American diet to a vegetarian or vegan diet. Take baby steps and allow your new habits to form.

Critical Success Factors for Healthy Earth Digestion

- Eliminate meat and dairy from your diet. Think of dairy as milk, yogurt, and cheese. Do not worry about the little bit of dairy found in cooked products.
- If you crave meat on occasion, consume it the way it is consumed in an Asian restaurant. Spice the meat and treat it as a condiment.
- Fall in love with pungent spices.
- Eat two to three meals each day around the same time each day. You can skip meals if you aren't hungry. Leave six hours between meals.
- Eat within one hour of rising.
- Lunch is your biggest meal.
- Foods are warm, dry, and cooked.
- No eating two to three hours before bedtime.
- No snacking.
- You benefit from a long walk after your meal.
- Favor foods in the following order:
  1. Beans. This is your staple.
  2. Cooked vegetables
  3. Whole grains. Quinoa is your best choice.
  4. Cooked fruits treated as dessert.
  5. Use very little nuts, seeds, honey, and oil. Use dry cooking methods like roasting and grilling.

6. Spice your foods up! This will make you feel satisfied. If you are normally a two at the Asian restaurant, start moving up the scale.

The following lists include items that your body type typically digests very well or not so well. Please eat consciously and simply notice if the foods aggravate you or appeal to you. Just because a food item appears on this list under avoid does not mean that you will be affected negatively by it. You have all the forces in your body; some other force may be helping you specifically to digest and enjoy items on the avoid side.

Notice that for fruits and vegetables, there is a theme: you are always choosing the lighter item. For example, if you were to simply pick up and hold a banana in one hand and an apple in the other, the apple would be the lighter fruit. The same is true for vegetables. Hold up a potato and some spinach. Obviously the spinach is lighter; it is your better choice.

Fruit:

Favor

All fruit except the heavy and dense fruits on the avoid list
Berries
Apples
Diluted fruit juice

Avoid

(heavy and dense)
Citrus fruits
Bananas
Melons
Avocado
Papaya

Vegetables:

Favor

Dark leafy greens
Spinach, kale, Swiss chard
Asparagus
Brussels sprouts
Mustard greens

Bok choy
Eggplant
Endives
Chicory
Romaine
Watercress
Okra

Avoid

Raw vegetables
Sweet potatoes
Squash
Cabbage
Parsnips
Corn
Carrots

Herbs that you can cook with or add to salads that are bitter include: Angelica, barberry, chamomile, dandelion, gentian, golden seal, milk thistle, mugwort, parsley, peppermint, tansy, and yarrow. Many of these are found in supplements and tea. The best bitter supplement is neem. You can take it daily to detoxify and improve digestion.

Beans and Legumes:

Favor

Mung beans
Lentils
Chickpeas

Avoid

(make your own avoid list)

I'm not going to place any bean on the avoid side. Try out all kinds of beans, as beans are your staple. Notice if the thicker-skinned beans create gas and bloating. If you can't spice them and cook them to avoid gas and bloating, then put them on your avoid list. More beans to try include adzuki, black, black-eyed peas, butter, cannellini, edamame, great northern, kidney, lima, navy, pinto, and soy.

Other:

Favor

Honey
All spices, especially pungent
All grains, except wheat and rice
Sunflower oil
All seeds
Wine

Avoid

All other sweeteners
All meat
All dairy
Anything the color white
Wheat and rice
Oil (use sparingly)
Nuts (use as a garnish only)
Beer and hard alcohol

The Earth loves amaranth, buckwheat, hempseed, soybeans, quinoa, and spirulina (take as a supplement) because they are complete proteins.

A Note from Pamela

People always ask me what I think they should take into their future from this Cleanse. First and foremost, never stop doing your work. The process of self-study and self-improvement never ends. As soon as you have conquered a situation, another will take its place. Embrace all of your experiences as opportunities to grow and learn.

I hope you love meditation and realize how wonderful it is for you. If you simply establish a meditation practice and do nothing else that I have recommended, your life will shift. It is truly powerful.

I hope you love yoga. Yoga is an amazing form of exercise appropriate for all bodies. It heals you on multiple levels. As you age you will find that your body simply can't endure some of our demanding exercise preferences. Yoga is a practice for a lifetime.

Every single day I take the following supplements: flaxseed oil, neem, and triphala (not the blend of triphala guggulu used in the Cleanse, just triphala). I do recommend that you stay on this herbal therapy for life.

Every single day I massage with sesame oil. I use it to take off my makeup. Once a week I soak my hair and sleep with oil in my hair. It will dynamically change the quality of your skin and reverse the aging process.

Take silence into your life. Give yourself a break from the media. The news really doesn't change all that much.

I drink the Yogi Breakfast pretty regularly. It keeps me from skipping breakfast.

I drink ginger tea every single day.

I wish that you would never drink cow's milk or eat red meat ever again.

I wish you would keep the Cleansing Dish as a side dish in your diet and consume it a few times each week.

You have a foundation to further your studies in Ayurveda and to begin to deeply learn about your dosha. I have provided an extended reading list of some of my favorite Ayurvedic books for you to enjoy. Ayurveda is dense and rich. It includes not just yoga, meditation, and nutrition but also aromatherapy, color therapy, marma point therapy, and astrology. There is even an Ayurvedic version of Feng Shui.

Never stop learning.

I wish you happiness, love and joy!

Shanti, Pamela

Supplemental Information and Recipes

Shopping List

Always stock these items in your pantry and refrigerator and you will always have a twenty-minute meal. Select organic, local, and whole.

Whole grain mixed rice
Whole grain pasta
Other whole grains such as barley, quinoa, oats, couscous
Whole grain bread, pita, pizza crust, and tortilla
Vegetable stock
Dried beans (choose beans that can be cooked in less than thirty minutes, including lentils, dahl, dal, mung, and split pea; *dahl* is Sanskrit for lentil)
Light coconut milk (in the can)
Curry paste
Organic pasta sauce and pizza sauce
Organic iodized sea salt
Pungent spices including peppers, cayenne, cumin, turmeric
Organic peanut butter, almond butter, or other
Soy, almond, rice, coconut, hemp, or hazelnut milk (sweetened or unsweetened)
Organic unsalted butter
Onion
Garlic
Ginger
Peppers
Carrots
Celery
Greens
Lemons

Dates
Nuts (your favorite) and dried fruit (your favorite, including figs/dates)

Every Sunday (or choose your cooking day), plan to make a big pot of rice and a big pot of bean-based soup. Separate and freeze in individual servings so it is ready to go for your week.

Cranberry Bliss Balls

Snack on Bliss Balls to your heart's content. You will find they are very rich and filling and hard to overindulge in.

1 cup sunflower seeds
1 cup almonds
2 cups dried cranberries
1 cup raisins
6–8 figs or dates, dried
2 tablespoons or more of maple syrup or honey
1 teaspoon vanilla extract
1 teaspoon or more nutmeg
½ cup shredded coconut flakes

Place all the nuts and dried fruit in a food processor and process until relatively smooth. Add the maple syrup, vanilla, and nutmeg. Continue to pulse until the mixture begins to stick together. Taste for sweetness. Add more maple syrup if necessary to hold the bliss balls together.

Place the shredded coconut flakes in a flat bowl. Roll the nut and cranberry mixture into one-inch balls, dip in maple syrup, and roll in the coconut flakes to coat. Store in an airtight container.

Play around with these. You may use any dried fruit or nut combination that you love. Consider figs, dates, raisins, and other nuts. You might also consider adding carob or a high-quality dark chocolate.

Digestive Aids

Ginger Elixir

Ginger supports healthy digestion and weight loss and is an integral part of The Elemental Cleanse.

How to Use: Take a small amount fifteen minutes or so prior to eating each meal. The ginger will act as a stimulant for your digestion. You may also place a small amount in hot water for a refreshing ginger tea.

Fresh ginger
Organic or sea salt
Fresh lemon or lime juice

Peel the ginger, then finely grate or slice the ginger into an airtight container. Add organic or sea salt to taste and cover with lemon or lime juice.

Place, sealed, in the refrigerator and gently shake the mixture once a day for three days. The marinated ginger will keep in the refrigerator for up to three weeks.

Lassi (Digestive Aid Smoothie)

Lassi is a yogurt drink that is to be used as a meal replacement. Various yogurts, juices, and spices can be used to create this delicious drink that is simply a blend of yogurt to liquid.

Organic plain yogurt or kefir
Water or fruit juice
Ginger
Organic salt
Cumin
Cilantro
Rosehips

Blend 40 percent yogurt and 60 percent water. Add spices as desired—ginger, salt, cumin, cilantro, and rosehips. You may consider using fruit juices such as mango instead of water. Play with the spices for balance of your Element.

Ghee or Clarified Butter

When unsalted butter is heated, it clarifies, or separates into three components: lactose or sugar, milk protein, and fat. The heat makes the moisture evaporate, the sugar and protein separate into the white curds that float or sink to the bottom. The leftover is pure, sweet, nutty, and yummy ghee. You can use ghee for frying, sautéing, or drizzling over veggies or grains.

Ghee is lactose free, easy to digest, heating and therefore a digestive aid. It increases Ojas, which is the sparkling divine essence that flows through you and nourishes you.

To make ghee, place 1 pound of unsalted organic butter in a heavy, medium-sized pan. Turn the heat to medium until the butter melts.

Turn down the heat until the butter just boils and continue to cook at this heat. Do not cover the pot. The butter will foam and sputter while it cooks. Whitish curds will begin to form on the bottom and top of the pot.

The butter will begin to smell like popcorn and will turn a lovely, golden color. Keep a close watch on the ghee, as it can easily burn. It will become a clear, golden color. Use a clean, dry spoon to move away some of the foam on top in order to see if the ghee is clear all the way through to the bottom.

When it is clear and has stopped sputtering and making noise, remove it from the heat. Let it cool until just warm. Pour it through a fine sieve or layers of cheesecloth into a clean, dry glass container with a tight lid. Discard the curds at the bottom of the saucepan.

The ghee is burned if it has a nutty smell and is slightly brown.

One pound of butter takes about fifteen minutes of cooking time. The more butter you are using, the more time the process will take.

The medicinal properties of ghee are said to improve with age. Don't ladle out the ghee with a wet spoon or allow any water to get into the container, as this will create conditions for bacteria to grow and spoil the ghee. Make sure the ghee is completely cooled before you put the lid on.

Two pounds of butter will fill a quart jar with ghee. Store ghee away from light and moisture and it will keep for up to twelve months without refrigeration.

Cleansing Dish

The Cleansing Dish (kitchari) can be eaten at any time, not just when you are on The Elemental Cleanse. There are many variations of the dish, so you can easily add it into your daily routine. This dish is very nutritious and easy to digest; it gives your digestive system a little break. This dish is especially good if you are experiencing any digestive disorders.

There are millions of variations of kitchari. It is basically India's staple food and is eaten daily there. You can also do a web search for kitchari to find more ideas.

To prepare the Cleansing Dish you'll need:

1 bag mung dal (If split, you do not have to soak. If whole, soak for an hour or even overnight. Mung dal or lentils are red, yellow, and green. The red dal tends to be more heating.)

Vegetable broth or water
Garlic, minced
Onion, chopped
Celery, chopped
Carrots, chopped
Organic salt and pepper, to taste
Cumin, 2 or more tablespoons
Cayenne pepper, to taste
White or brown rice, prefer basmati (see note below)

Always rinse your beans before cooking and remove any discolored beans. Place mung dal in pot and cover with vegetable broth. Bring to boil and then reduce to simmer. Add garlic, onions, celery, carrots, salt, pepper, cumin, and cayenne pepper. Simmer on low until beans are cooked through. You may cover with a lid. You will have to keep checking the liquid level and adding broth or water to keep moist. This should take forty minutes or so.

You may add the rice to your pot and cook all as one or cook the rice separately.

Note on rice: Serve with brown rice for daily consumption or white rice if you are resting your digestion or performing the last week of The Elemental Cleanse.

Variations to make the Cleansing Dish recipe unique to you:

- Even when using broth, it is nice to throw in some organic mushroom bouillon cubes. These really give a blast of flavor.
- **Don't be afraid of spice**. Add everything to taste. You may want to double the amount of cumin you use. Try other spices as well.
- **All veggies are good in this.** You can add peas, spinach, kale, or potatoes. Anything you have in your refrigerator will do.
- If you want even more **flavor**, sauté your veggies in ghee before you add them to the pot.
- If you want a **soupier soup**, add more broth. If you want a denser meal, let the water simmer off.
- If you want **crunchier lentils**, don't cook as long.
- If you want a **richer kitchari**, pour some coconut milk in.
- If you want to **turn this into a breakfast treat**, make the following changes. Instead of veggies, use dried fruit like raisins. Instead of peppery spices, use sweet spices like nutmeg and cinnamon. Add a little ghee and honey and you have breakfast (you can always add coconut milk too).

Yogi Breakfast

This breakfast is perfect for all yogis. It is sattvic, which means it contains only pure ingredients that are easy to digest. You may use milk, soymilk, almond milk, or rice milk. For The Earth (Kapha), it is suggested to not use cow's milk.

8 almonds
1 cup milk, soymilk, almond milk, or rice milk
1 teaspoon honey
Nutmeg
Cinnamon
Ginger (optional)

Place the almonds in the bottom of a small pan. Pour the milk over and heat on low until milk is warm and bubbles just on the edge. Remove from heat and poor in a mug. Add honey, nutmeg, and cinnamon to taste. Enjoy!

Breakfast Dahl

Beans for breakfast? You bet. This bean dish is better than oatmeal and will give you a great sweet start to your day.

1 cup dahl (I choose the smallest lightest color for this)
2 cans light coconut milk
2 Granny Smith apples
1/4 cup dried fruit of your choice (raisins, cranberries, prunes, plums)
1/4 cup organic brown sugar
2 tablespoons diced ginger
2 cloves diced garlic (that's right!)
Juice of one lime
1 tablespoon turmeric
Salt to taste
Cinnamon to taste

Put all ingredients in a small pot on the stove together. Bring to a boil. Cover and reduce to simmer. Check on it occasionally for the next thirty minutes, adding more coconut milk as needed. If you want to turn this into a complete protein, simply add one cup of rice and two more cups of liquid.

Additional Recommended Reading

Heaven's Banquet by Miriam Kasin Hospodar
Ayurveda and Panchakarma: The Science of Healing Rejuvenation by Dr. Sunhil, M.D.
Ayurveda and Aromatherapy: Earth Essential Guide to Ancient Wisdom and Modern Healing by Dr. Light Miller and Dr. Bryan Miller
The Yoga of Herbs by Dr. Vasant Lad
The Complete Book of Ayurvedic Home Remedies by Dr. Vasant Lad
The Ayurvedic Cookbook by Amandea Morningstar
Perfect Digestion by Deepak Chopra

Made in the USA
Lexington, KY
16 February 2019